Faecal incontinence
and related problems
in the older adult

This book is dedicated to my wife Pauline and
and children Anthony, Maria, Michael, Cassandra
and Lucinda

FAECAL INCONTINENCE AND RELATED PROBLEMS IN THE OLDER ADULT

J.A. BARRETT MD, MRCP
Consultant Physician in Geriatric Medicine,
Clatterbridge Hospital, Wirral

Edward Arnold
A division of Hodder & Stoughton
LONDON BOSTON MELBOURNE AUCKLAND

© 1993 James A. Barrett

First published in Great Britain 1993
Distributed in the Americas by Little, Brown and Company
34 Beacon Street, Boston, MA 02108

British Library Cataloguing in Publication Data

Barrett, James A.
  Faecal incontinence and related problems
  in the older adult
  I. Title
  618.97

  ISBN 0–340–54361–2

Typeset in 10/11 Palatino by Anneset, Weston-super-Mare, Avon.
Printed in Great Britain for Edward Arnold, a division of Hodder and Stoughton Limited, Mill Road, Dunton Green, Sevenoaks, Kent TN13 2YA by St. Edmundsbury Press, Bury St. Edmunds, Suffolk.
Bound by Hartnolls Ltd, Bodmin, Cornwall.

Foreword

It has been observed of urinary incontinence that, although it is rarely fatal, it may bring social death. And this is even more true of faecal incontinence. It would be difficult to exaggerate the distress that it may cause – not only for the sufferer but also for carers. This is in part due to physical discomfort but also to the intense embarrassment and feeling of humiliation that may accompany it. Even the fear of incontinence may lead to severe curtailment of social activities and a dramatic shrinkage of life-space. The onset of incontinence is often the final straw that causes breakdown of home care.

For this reason, *Faecal Incontinence and Related Problems in the Older Adult* is especially welcome. Its author, Dr. James Barrett, is a consultant geriatrician. He did his MD research under the direction of Professor John Brocklehurst and it is not surprising, therefore, that this book is in the Brocklehurst tradition: it effortlessly encompasses all aspects of the complex problem of faecal incontinence from the pathophysiological to the social, combining a high level of clinical science with an excellent exposition of the practical details of good multidisciplinary care. The result of this multi-levelled and multi-faceted approach is a superbly authoritative and comprehensive text. Although the detailed account of ano-rectal physiology and colonic motility and the influence upon this of factors such as ageing will make this book an ideal reference for experts and those embarking on research in the field, *Faecal Incontinence and Related Problems in the Older Adult* is also full of carefully argued advice on practical management. The account of the rational use of laxatives, of the approach to overflow incontinence and of the management of diarrhoea – to take only three examples – are models of clarity. This text will therefore find a place not only in research units but wherever professionals are trained in the medical care of the elderly and wherever patients are cared for – in hospital wards, in nursing homes and in the community.

The good news about faecal incontinence in the elderly is that, with appropriate management, patients can, in the majority of cases, regain control over their bowels and in the remaining cases the problem can be greatly alleviated. The rigorous science and good clinical sense in this book should ensure that appropriate management is more widespread. It is a pleasure to commend what looks like being a major contribution to the literature dealing with 'the giants of geriatric medicine'.

R. Tallis
University Professor of Geriatric Medicine
Hope Hospital

Preface

This book, *Faecal Incontinence and Related Problems in the Older Adult*, has been written principally for medical and nursing staff working with elderly people with or without disabilities.

The content of this book is also relevant for professionals working with younger people with disabilities or with terminal disease as they often experience the same bowel problems that are common in the elderly, i.e. constipation and faecal incontinence.

Previous books on this subject have concentrated on the surgical approach to the management of faecal incontinence in young and middle-aged patients.

This is the first book to concentrate mainly on the problems experienced by older patients in whom the prevalence is highest and who require a different management approach.

Normal anorectal physiology, ageing effects and the pathophysiology of anorectal incontinence are discussed in the first section of the book. The main causes of faecal incontinence are dealt with in the second section followed by discussion of the practical management of faecal incontinence, constipation and other related problems. The psychological aspects of faecal incontinence are included for the first time in a book on faecal incontinence.

Acknowledgements

I wish to acknowledge the support and encouragement that I received from Professor J.C. Brocklehurst and Mr. E.S. Kiff during the research sutdies that I performed at the University Hospital of South Manchester, Margaret Blakeborough for her practical assistance during the research studies; the numerous patients who consented to the studies;

Carol Hart, Maureen Fanning and Anna Banks (Continence Advisors) for their assistance in devising methods of managing intractable faecal incontinence; and finally, Professor Ray Tallis for his encouragement during the preparation of this manuscript.

Contributors

Linda J. Smith Clinical Psychologist, Rehabilitation Northern Trust, Sanderson Centre, Gosforth, Newcastle-upon-Tyne

Paul S. Smith Clinical Psychologist, Northumberland Psychology Services, Northgate Hospital, Morpeth, Northumberland

Contents

Foreword   **v**

Preface   **vii**

List of contributors   **ix**

1. Introduction   **1**

2. Anatomy of the Colon, Rectum and Anus   **3**
Higher control of defaecation   3
The colon   3
Rectum and anus   5

3. Assessment of Anal Function   **12**
Anal manometry   12
Recto-anal inhibitory reflex   14
Electromyography   15

4. Maintenance of anal continence   **18**
Anal sphincter pressure zone   18
Reflex activity   21
Puborectalis muscle and the anorectal angle   22
Anorectal sensation and the sampling reflex   22
Rectal sensation   24
Slit shaped anal canal and mechanical factors   25
Vascular and mucosal component   25

5. Normal Defaecation   **29**
Gut transit   29
Colonic activity   30
Rectal activity   32
The act of defaecation   36

 6. **Anorectal Incontinence (Idiopathic Faecal Incontinence)**   **40**
    Direct injury to the anal sphincter   40
    External anal sphincter and pelvic floor muscle weakness   41
    Obstetric factors   43
    Perineal descent (descending perineum syndrome)   46
    Rectal prolapse   47
    Effect of disease of the spinal cord or cauda equina   47
    Ageing and anorectal incontinence   47
    Anorectal sensory loss   47
    Internal sphincter weakness   49
    Diabetes   52
    Multiple sclerosis   52
    Spinal cord disease or injury   53

 7. **Ageing and Anorectal Function**   **60**
    Ageing and bowel habit   60
    The effect of age on anal resting pressure   61
    The effect of age on the external anal sphincter and
    its innervation   61
    Ageing and the recto-anal reflex   65
    The effect of age on rectal sensation   65
    Ageing and defaecation   67
    Ageing and anal sensation   67

 8. **Faecal Incontinence in the Elderly – Introduction**   **70**

 9. **Anorectal Function of Elderly Patients with Faecal
    Incontinence**   **71**
    External anal sphincter function   71
    Internal anal sphincter dysfunction   72
    Anal sensation   74

10. **Symptomatic Faecal Incontinence and Its Management**   **76**
    Colorectal tumours   76
    Infective diarrhoea   78
    Inflammatory bowel disease   79
    Bile acid diarrhoea   83

11. **Idiopathic Constipation**   **86**
    Colonic motility/transit   86
    Defaecatory difficulty   91
    Rectal sensation   93
    Urological problems in constipation   94
    Megarectum   94
    Gynaecological problems in constipation   95
    Constipation and haemorrhoids   96
    Psychiatric symptoms in constipation   96
    Drug induced constipation   97

12. Constipation in the Elderly **101**
Diagnosis 101
Definition 102
Pathophysiology of constipation 103

13. Faecal Incontinence Secondary to Constipation **110**
Anal manometry 110
Stool consistency 111
Anorectal angle 111
Rectal sensation 111
Anal sensation 112
Laxative induced faecal incontinence 112
Conclusion 112

14. Faecal Incontinence Secondary to Cerebral Disease **114**
Impaired consciousness 114
Patients with dementing illnesses 114
Stroke 121
Parkinson's disease 122

15. Faecal Incontinence in the Elderly – Overview **124**

**16. Clinical Assessment of the Faecally Incontinent Elderly
Patient** **129**
The history 129
Physical examination 130
Investigations 131

17. Treatment of Faecal Incontinence – Introduction **133**

18. Treatment of Faecal Incontinence Secondary to Faecal Loading **135**
Initial treatment of the incontinent faecally loaded patient 135
Treatment of faecal loading which fails to respond to initial
treatment 137
Prevention of recurrence 139
Biofeedback in the treatment of constipation 144
Surgical management of constipation 144
Spinal stimulators 145

19. Treatment of Diarrhoea **150**

**20. Treatment of Faecal Incontinence Secondary to Cerebral
Disease** **153**

21. Treatment of Anorectal Incontinence **157**
Biofeedback 157
Electrical stimulation 159
Surgical treatment 161

22. Treatment of Intractable Faecal Incontinence **168**

23. Psychological Aspects of Faecal Incontinence in the Elderly
Linda J. Smith and Paul S. Smith   **173**
Introduction   173
The personal and emotional experience of being incontinent   174
Personality, mental health and faecal incontinence   175
Psychological approaches to the treatment of faecal
incontinence   177
General environmental effects   179
The psycho-analytic approach   182
Behavioural approaches to treatment   182
Other factors in training programmes   185
Continence training specifically with the elderly or
elderly confused   189
Other psychological approaches: anxiety reduction   200

Index   **207**

1

Introduction

Faecal incontinence is a distressing problem that may occur at any age after bowel control is achieved but is most prevalent in elderly people living in institutions.

In a large community survey, Thomas *et al.* (1985) estimated that the community prevalence of faecal incontinence occurring at least twice per month is four per 1000 in men and two per 1000 in women aged 15–64 years and 11 per 1000 in men and 13 per 1000 in women aged over 65 years. This represents approximately 1000 people in a district with a population of 250,000.

These results illustrate that the problem of faecal incontinence is most prevalent among the elderly. It is surprising that the strong female bias that is generally recognised in the younger patients in clinical practice was not detected in this study.

Seventy-two percent of the elderly incontinent patients in Thomas *et al.*'s study were living in institutions. Of those living at home only 16% were fully mobile, 35% were incontinent at least once per day and 20% had been incontinent for at least five years.

Kok *et al.* (1992), in a community based study in The Netherlands have demonstrated that within the elderly age group there is a significant increase in the prevalence of faecal incontinence (defined as occasional faecal leakage) with increasing age from less than 4% in the under-75s up to 16% in nonagenarians.

Faecal incontinence is poorly tolerated by the families caring for debilitated elderly patients at home and its onset frequently leads to a request for admission to a geriatric unit (Sanford 1975). Faecal incontinence is the problem that carers are least able to tolerate. It is therefore suprising to find that faecal incontinence is often taken for granted by staff caring for patients in institutions when effective treatment is available (Tobin and Brocklehurst 1986).

Major advances have been made in understanding why faecal incontinence occurs and how to manage it. Most of the physiological studies have been performed on younger patients but information is now also available about the problem in the elderly. The main emphasis in this book is on the problems of faecal incontinence and constipation in the elderly. Extensive reference is made to the research which has been carried out on young and middle aged patients with these problems. Lower gastrointestinal problems which are associated with faecal incontinence are also discussed.

References

Kok ALM, Voorhorst FJ, Burger CW, Van Houten P, Kenemans P, Janssens J. (1992) Urinary and faecal incontinence in commmunity-residing elderly women. *Age and Ageing*; **21**: 211–15.

Sanford JRA. (1975) Tolerance of debility in elderly dependants by supporters at home: its significance for hospital practice. *Br. Med. J*; **3**: 471–3.

Thomas TM, Egan M, Meade TW. (1985) Prevalence and implications of faecal (and double) incontinence. *Br. J. Surg.*; **72** Supplement: S141.

Tobin GW, Brocklehurst JC. (1986) Faecal incontinence in residential homes for the elderly: prevalence, aetiology and management. *Age and Ageing*; **15**: 41–46.

2

Anatomy of the colon, rectum and anus

The main function of the colon, rectum and anus is the acceptance of undigested liquid material from the small bowel, the absorption of water from that material, the storage and retention of the faecal material that results from the above and the defaecation of that material in a socially acceptable place.

Higher control of defaecation

Normal faecal continence and defaecation are social skills that are achieved during the first two to three years of life with the establishment of a higher centre to control defaecation (Howard and Nixon, 1968). Andrew and Nathan (1964, 1965) following their study of patients with lesions of the forebrain, suggested that the total acts of defaecation and micturition are organised in the hypothalamus and that the integration of defaecation and micturition into normal daily activities within the environment is centred in the superior frontal gyrus and the anterior part of the cingulate gyrus.

   Most of the activity of the colon, rectum and anus occurs without any voluntary control. Complex mechanisms control their activity. These are still to be fully elucidated but many of the basic principles are understood.

The colon

The colon (Fig. 1) is a 1.5 metre long hollow tube which extends from the ileocaecal valve to the rectum. Its wall consists of four main layers

– mucosa, submucosa, inner circular and outer longitudinal muscle layers and a serosal covering. The nerve supply of the colon is derived from sympathetic and parasympathetic nerves and two nerve plexuses – the myenteric plexus which lies between the circular and longitudinal muscle layers and the submucous plexus (Williams and Warwick, 1980; Wyburn, 1972).

Nerve supply of the colon and rectum

The motor control of the colon and rectum is under the control of a number of mechanisms which include splanchnic nerves, enteric nerves and hormonal systems.

The vagus nerve innervates the right colon to its midportion, with the parasympathetic innervation of the distal colon being mainly derived from pelvic parasympathetic nerves. The vagus nerve has a stimulatory effect upon the proximal colon with some effect also on the distal colon (Hulten and Jodal, 1969, Esser *et al.*, 1989). This response is readily blocked by atropine, indicating a cholinergic response (Hulten and Jodal 1969).

Burleigh (1990) has demonstrated *in vitro* that human circular colonic muscle strips exhibit a high degree of spontaneous activity with regular contractions and relaxtions. Longitudinal muscle activity was less predictable and less spontaneous. Acetylcholine was found to contract human colonic muscle strips.

Sympathetic innervation of the colon and rectum is derived from the lumbar colonic nerves and hypogastric nerves. The colonic innervation is considered to be mostly inhibitory (Hulten, 1969) but there may be a

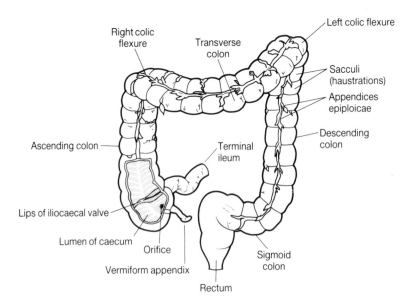

Fig. 1   Diagrams of the colon.

stimulatory sympathetic effect upon the rectum as epidural anaesthesia has been shown to increase rectal tone (Carlstedt *et al.*, 1988). Noradrenaline has been found to produce colonic muscle contraction (Burleigh, 1990).

Normal motility of the colon is dependent upon the enteric nervous system which has been described as the 'gut brain'. The myenteric and submucous plexuses form an important part of this, with fibres supplying muscle mucosa and blood vessels, and they have interconnecting fibres. Milner et al (1990) have demonstrated that myenteric plexus cell bodies contain vasoactive peptide (VIP), substance *P* and neuropeptide Y, and that VIP containing nerve cell bodies project to the circular muscle, the submucous plexus and distally to other cell bodies within the myenteric plexus. VIP was found by Grider *et al.* (1985) to have an inhibitory effect on peristalsis. Burleigh (1990) has shown that VIP causes contraction of circular colonic muscle which is more marked in the distal colon and that the longitudinal muscle is comparatively insensitive to VIP.

Substance *P* has an excitatory effect on peristalsis (Bartho and Holzer 1985; Goldin *et al.*, 1989).

Rectum and anus

The rectum (Fig. 2) begins in contact with the pelvic surface of the third sacral vertebra as a continuation of the sigmoid colon. Its lumen becomes the anal canal as it passes downwards and posteriorly surrounded by the internal and external anal sphincters. The anal canal is 2.5 to 5cm in length and 3cm in diameter when distended. The axis of the rectum forms almost a right angle (average 82°) with the axis of the anal canal (Hardcastle and Parks, 1970). The former concept of the anal

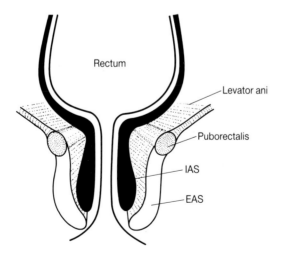

Fig. 2 Anteroposterior view of anus and rectum.

canal being surrounded successively by internal anal sphincter and then the external anal sphincter has been replaced by the knowledge that the two muscles overlap to a considerable extent with the external sphincter wrapped around the internal sphincter (Goligher *et al.*, 1955; Lawson, 1970).

The circular smooth muscle of the rectum is continued into the internal anal sphincter (Fig. 3) which is 1.5 to 5mm in thickness and surrounds the proximal 2–4cm of the anal canal. Fibrous extensions of the outer longitudinal coat of the rectum interdigitate with the levator ani and external anal sphincter muscles.

The levator ani muscles form the pelvic floor and their most important component in maintaining anal continence is the puborectalis muscle which arises from the posterior aspect of the pubis, inferior to the pubococcygeus, and passes posteriorly around the anorectal junction to join with the puborectalis from the other side to form a sling. Contraction of this muscle sling pulls the anorectal junction upwards and forwards and increases the angle between the anus and rectum (anorectal angle) (see Fig. 3).

The external anal sphincter surrounds the distal 2–3cm of the internal anal sphincter and projects for 0.5–1cm distal to it. It is attached to the perineal body anteriorly and to the coccyx posteriorly.

Nerve supply of pelvic floor and anus

The pelvic floor and external anal sphincter muscles are innervated mainly by the pudendal nerve and its branches.

The pudendal nerve arises in the pelvis from the second, third and

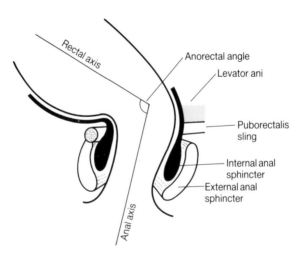

Fig. 3 Lateral view of the anus and rectum demonstrating normal anal resting and squeeze pressures.

fourth sacral nerve roots. It passes through the greater sciatic notch close to the ischial spine, and enters the perineum through the pudendal canal on the obturator fascia of the lateral wall of the ischiorectal fossa. Here it gives off the inferior rectal nerve and shortly afterwards divides into the perineal nerve and the dorsal nerve of the penis or clitoris. The inferior rectal nerve supplies the external anal sphincter muscle and receives sensory fibres from the anus and perianal skin (Wyburn, 1972; Kiff 1984).

The levator ani is supplied by a branch from the fourth sacral spinal nerve and by a branch which arises from either the inferior rectal nerve or from the perineal division of the pudendal nerve (Williams and Warwick, 1980). Its nerve supply is separate from that of the external sphincter (Matzel *et al.*, 1990).

The nerve supply to puborectalis is from sacral motor nerves derived from the S3 and S4 nerve roots and is separate from that to the external sphincter (Percy *et al.*, 1981; Snooks *et al.*, 1985).

Nerve supply of the internal anal sphincter

The internal anal sphincter is controlled by both extrinsic autonomic pathways and intrinsic enteric nerves. The autonomic innervation is from sympathetic nerves derived from the inferior hypogastric plexus and parasympathetic nerves from the second, third and fourth sacral segments of the spinal cord.

a) Sympathetic

Direct high frequency peroperative stimulation of the presacral sympathetic nerves has been shown to produce relaxation of the internal sphincter (Shepherd and Wright, 1968; Lubowski *et al.*, 1987; Carlstedt *et al*, 1988) though Frenckner and Ihre (1976) inferred from their study of anal sphincter tone during spinal anaesthesia at high and low thoracolumbar levels that the sympathetic innervation of the internal anal sphincter had an excitatory effect.

In vitro tests on isolated strips of human internal anal sphincter muscle have shown it to contract in response to noradrenaline (Kerremans, 1969; Friedman, 1968; Parks *et al.*, 1969) and relax in response to isoprenaline. The effect of adrenaline varied, with low concentrations producing relaxation and contraction with high concentrations.

Parks *et al.* (1969) explained this observation by proposing that the internal sphincter smooth muscle contains alpha adrenergic receptors subserving contraction and beta receptors subserving relaxation. The conversion of noradrenergic contraction of internal sphincter muscle strips into relaxation activity by alpha-adrenoreceptor antagonists supports this proposal (Friedman, 1968; Parks *et al.*, 1969).

Beta-adrenergic relaxation of the internal sphincter has been produced by isoprenaline infusion in human volunteers, an effect that can be blocked by propranolol (Gutierrez and Shah, 1975).

b) Parasympathetic

Meunier and Mollard (1977) suggested that the internal sphincter was dependent upon a stimulatory parasympathetic nerve supply as they found that anal sphincter resting tone was reduced in meningocoele patients who are theoretically devoid of parasympathetic pathways but who have a normal sympathetic outflow.

The parasympathetic neurotransmitter acetylcholine has, however, been shown to relax strips of internal sphincter muscle *in vitro* (Burleigh *et al.*, 1979) which confirms the *in vivo* observation that bethanecol (parasympathomimetic) lowers anal canal resting pressure (Gutierrez and Shah, 1975). The effect of bethanecol can be blocked by atropine which causes a small increase in anal tone (Gutierrez and Shah, 1975).

c) Enteric nervous system

Burleigh *et al.* (1979) demonstrated that the internal sphincter receives an innervation from the enteric nervous system consisting of non- cholinergic, non-cathecolaminergic nerves which may utilise purinergic or peptidergic transmitters.

In summary, the autonomic control of the internal anal sphincter appears to be mediated through complex alpha-excitatory and beta-inhibitory adrenergic pathways with probable inhibitory cholinergic pathways and non-adrenergic, non-cholinergic pathways. The net balance between these excitatory and inhibitory influences determines internal sphincter tone.

The distribution of the regulatory neuropeptides VIP, substance P, Somatostatin, NPY, mammalian bombesin and substance PYY in the human sigmoid-recto-anal region is not uniform (Ferri *et al.*, 1988).

Anal sensation

The anal canal is sensitive to light touch, pressure, pain and temperature and is plentifully supplied with several types of specialised nerve endings (Duthie and Gairns, 1960; Holmes, 1961).

Rectal sensation

The rectum is insensitive to touch, pressure and temperature but is sensitive to distension which is interpreted as a call to stool (Duthie and Gairns, 1960). This sensation has been shown to increase as the anus is approached (Goligher and Hughes 1951). However, no organised nerve endings have been found in the rectum to subserve this sensation though there are numerous free nerve endings in the submucosa (Duthie and Gairns, 1960).

It has been suggested that rectal distension is sensed in the pelvic floor muscles, as relatively normal sensation of rectal distension has been found in the colon of patients after low anterior resection (Goligher and Hughes, 1951; Suzuki *et al.*, 1980; Williams *et al.*, 1980), rectal excision and colo-anal anastomosis (Lane and Parks, 1977; Parks and Percy, 1982) and in the neorectum of patients after proctocolectomy and ileal pouch formation (Parks *et al.*, 1980). Muscle spindles have been found in levator ani (Winckler, 1958) and the external sphincter (Parks *et al.*, 1977; Walls, 1959) which could subserve this sensation. Stretch of the puborectalis has also been proposed as the possible stimulus responsible for the desire to defaecate (Varma and Stephens, 1972; Scharli and Kiesewetter, 1970; Parks, 1975).

It seems probable, though, that more than one pathway subserves rectal sensation in the normal subject as rectal sensation is unaffected by block of the nerve supply to the external sphincter and puborectalis (Frenckner and Euler, 1975) but is lost after section of the parasympathetic pelvic nerves (Goligher and Hughes, 1951).

References

Andrew J, Nathan PW. (1964) Lesions of the anterior frontal lobes and disturbances of micturition and defaecation. *Brain*; **87**: 233–62.

Andrew J, Nathan PW. (1965) The cerebral control of micturition. *Proc Roy Soc Med*; **58**: 553–5.

Bartho L, Holzer P. (1985) Search for a physiological role for substance P in gastrointestinal motility. *Neuroscience*; **16**: 1–32.

Burleigh DE. (1990) Motor responsiveness of proximal and distal human colonic muscle layers to acetylcholine, noradrenaline, and vasoactive intestinal peptide. *Digestive Diseases and Sciences*; **35**: 617–21.

Burleigh DE, D'mello A, Parks AG (1970) Response of isolated human internal anal spincter to drugs and electrical held stimulation. *Gastroenterology*; **77**: 484–490.

Carlstedt A, Nordgren S, Fasth S, Appelgren L, Hulten L. (1988) Sympathetic nervous influence on the internal anal sphincter and rectum in man. *Int J Colorectal Dis*; **3**: 90–5.

Duthie HL, Gairns FW. (1960) Sensory nerve endings and sensation in the anal region of man. *Br J Surg*; **206**: 585–94.

Esser MJ, Cowles VE, Robinson JC, Schulte WJ, Gleysteen JJ, Condon RE. (1989) Effects of vagal cryo-interruption on colon contractions in monkeys. *Surgery*; **106**: 139–46.

Ferri GL, Adrian TE, Allen JM, *et al. (1988) Intramural distribution of regulatory peptides in the sigmoid-recto-anal region of the human gut. Gut.* **29**: 762–8.

Frenckner B, Euler CV. (1975) Influence of pudendal nerve block on the function of the anal sphincters. *Gut*; **16**: 482–9.

Frenckner B, Ihre T. (1976) Influence of the autonomic nerves on the internal anal sphincter in man. *Gut*; **17**: 306–12.

Friedman CA. (1968) The action of nicotine and catecholamines on the human internal anal sphincter. *Am J Dig Dis*; **13**: 428–31.

Goldin E, Karmeli F, Selinger Z, Rachmilewitz D. (1989) Colonic substance P levels are increased in ulcerative colitis and decreased in chronic severe constipation. *Dig Dis Sci*; **34**: 754–7.

Goligher JC, Hughes ESR. (1951) Sensibility of the rectum and colon: its role in the mechanism of anal continence. *Lancet*; **i**: 543–8.

Goligher JC, Leacock AG, Brossy JJ. (1955) The surgical anatomy of the anal canal. *Br J Surg*; **43**: 51–61.

Grider JR, Cable MB, Bitar KN, Said SI, Makhlouf GM. (1985). Vasoactive intestinal peptide. Relaxant neurotransmitter in taenia coli of the guinea pig. *Gastroenterology*; **89**: 36–42.

Gutierrez JG, Shah AN. (1975). Autonomic control of the internal anal sphincter in man. In van Trappen G (ed) Fifth International Symposium of Gastrointestinal Motility, pp. 363–73. Typoff Press, Belgium.

Hardcastle JD, Parks AG. (1970). A study of anal incontinence and some principles of surgical treatment. *Proc Roy Soc Med*; **63**: 116–8.

Holmes AM. (1961) Observations of the intrinsic innervation of the rectum and anal canal. *J Anat*; **95**: 416–22.

Howard ER, Nixon HH. (1968). Internal anal sphincter. Observations on development and mechanisms of inhibitory responses in premature infants and children with Hirschsprung's disease. *Arch Dis Childhood*; **43**: 569–78.

Hulten L. (1969) Extrinsic nervous control of colonic motility and blood flow. *Acta Physiol Scand* (Suppl); **335**: 1–116.

Hulten L, Jodal M. (1969) Extrinsic nervous control of colonic motility. *Acta Physiol Scand* (Suppl); **335**: 21–38.

Kerremans R. (1969) *Morphological and Physiological Aspects of Anal Continence and Defaecation*. Editions Arsica, Brussels.

Kiff ES. (1984) Studies of ano-rectal physiology in relation to the aetiology of idiopathic faecal incontinence. MD thesis, Manchester University.

Lane RHS, Parks AG. (1977) Function of the anal sphincters following colo- anal anastomosis. *Br J Surg*; **64**: 596–9.

Lawson JON. (1970) Structure and function of the internal anal sphincter. *Proc Roy Soc Med*; **63** (Suppl): 84–9.

Lubowski DZ, Nicholls RJ, Swash M, Jordan MJ. (1987) Neural control of internal anal sphincter function. *Br J Surg*; **74**: 668–70.

Matzel KE, Schmidt RA, Tanagho EA. (1990) Neuroanatomy of the striated muscular anal continence mechanism. Implications for the use of neurostimulation. *Dis Colon Rectum*; **33**: 666–73.

Meunier P, Mollard P. (1977) Control of the internal anal sphincter (manometric study with human subjects). *Pflugers Archiv*; **370**: 233–9.

Milner P, Crowe R, Kamm MA, Lennard-Jones JE, Burnstock G. (1990) Vasoactive polypeptide in sigmoid colon in idiopathic constipation and diverticular disease. *Gastroenterology*; **99**: 666–75.

Parks AG. (1975) Anorectal incontinence. *Proc Roy Soc Med*; **68**: 681–90.

Parks AG, Fishlock DJ, Cameron JDH, May H. (1969) Preliminary investigation of the pharmacology of the human internal anal sphincter. *Gut*; **10** 674–7.

Parks AG, Nicholls RJ, Belliveau P. (1980). Proctocolectomy with ileal reservoir and anal anastomosis. *Br J Surg*; **67**: 533–8.

Parks AG, Percy JP. (1982) Resection and sutured colo-anal anastomosis for rectal carcinoma. *Br J Surg*; **69**: 301–4.

Parks AG, Swash M, Urich H. (1977) Sphincter denervation in anorectal incontinence and rectal prolapse. *Gut*; **18**: 656–65.

Percy JP, Neill ME, Swash M, Parks AG. (1981) Electrophysiological study of motor nerve supply of the pelvic floor. *Lancet*; **i**: 16–17.

Scharli AF, Kiesewetter WB. (1970). Defaecation and continence: some new concepts. *Dis Colon Rectum*; **13**: 81–107.

Shepherd JJ, Wright PG. (1968) The response of the internal anal sphincter in man to stimulation of the presacral nerve. *Am J Dig Dis*; **13**: 421–7.

Snooks SJ, Henry MM, Swash M. (1985) Anorectal incontinence and rectal prolapse: differential assessment of the innervation to puborectalis and external anal sphincter muscles. Gut; **26**: 470–6.

Suzuki H, Matsumuto K, Amano S, Fujioka M, Honzumi M. (1980) Anorectal pressure and rectal compliance after low anterior resection. Br J Surg; **67**: 655–7.

Varma KK, Stephens D. (1972) Neuromuscular reflex of rectal continence. *Aust NZ J Surg*; **41**: 252–63.

Walls EW. (1959) Recent observations on the anatomy of the anal canal. *Proc Roy Soc Med*; **52** (Suppl): 85–7.

Williams NS, Price R, Johnston D. (1980) The long term effects of sphincter preserving operations for rectal carcinoma on function of the anal sphincter in man. *Br J Surg*; **67**: 203–8.

Williams PL, Warwick R. (1980) *Grays Anatomy*, 36th edn. Churchill Livingstone, Edinburgh.

Winckler G. (1958) Remarques sur la morphologie et l'innervation du muscle releveur de l'anus. *Archives d'Anatomie, d'Histologie et d'Embryologie (Strasbourg)*; **41**: 77–95.

Wyburn GM. (1972) The digestive system. In Romanes GJ (ed) *Cunningham's Textbook of Anatomy*, pp. 399–467. Oxford Medical Publications, Oxford.

3

Assessment of anal function

In order to understand the anatomical and physiological mechanisms contribute towards the maintainence of continence it is necessary to understand the basic principles about the methods that are used to assess anal function. These are described in this chapter and supplemented with information in later chapters about more specialised techniques particularly in the investigation and study of faecal incontinence.

Anal manometry

Several methods are available for measuring anal canal pressure and these have been reviewed by Dickinson (1978). Most of the published studies in which anal manometry has been performed have used either an open-tipped catheter or a balloon system connected via a transducer to a chart recording system. Open tipped catheters have the disadvantage of becoming blocked with faeces. Erroneous values may be obtained when tubes with side openings are used as the anal canal is not a perfect cylinder (Kerremans, 1969). Continuous water perfusion of open-tipped catheters keeps them patent but this requires an expensive pump to maintain a constant rate of perfusion and the flow of water may irritate the anal and perianal skin and influence sphincter activity (Kerremans, 1969). Hancock (1976) also found that the rate of water perfusion influenced the measured pressure.

Covering the end of a water-filled catheter with an elastic balloon prevents its blockage by faeces. Henry and Parks (1980) demonstrated this system to be reliable. The balloons used have varied from 3mm to 15mm in diameter. The pressure recorded, however, varies with the diameter of the balloon (Hill *et al.*, 1960) or the catheter (McHugh and Diamant, 1987).

Miller *et al.*, (1989) have described an air filled microballoon manometry system which can be used as an alternative to the above methods.

Irrespective of the measuring device, most centres employ a pull through technique with the measurement of anal pressure at 0·5–1cm intervals to assess maximum anal resting pressure and maximum voluntary anal contraction (or anal squeeze) pressure (Fig 4).

Patients with abnormal anal sphincters demonstrated a deficiency of either resting pressure (Fig. 5) or squeeze pressure. In some patients a combined deficiency was identified (Fig. 6).

Strain gauge systems which measure radial force have also been devised but although they are reliable, they are difficult and expensive to construct and tend to be rather fragile (Collins *et al.*, 1967; Wankling *et al.*, 1968; Collins *et al.*, 1969). They are not in routine use.

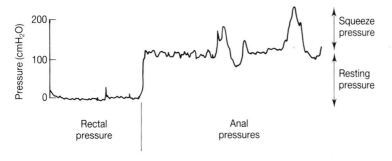

Fig. 4 Anorectal manometry trace demonstrating normal anal resting and squeeze pressures.

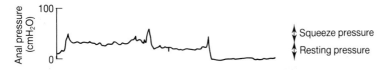

Fig. 5 Anorectal manometry trace demonstrating low anal resting pressure but normal squeeze pressure. A cough artefact is also demonstrated.

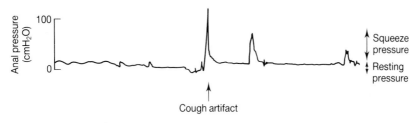

Fig. 6 Anorectal manometry trace demonstrating low anal resting and squeeze pressures.

Microtransducers, however, have the advantage of being smaller and are less likely to produce the artefacts which are expected with water filled systems. Microtransducers can be fitted into fine tubing in such a way as to allow ambient pressure to be conducted via a plastic membrane to an ultra-thin metal diaphragm, which is in turn connected to a strain gauge (Miller *et al.*, 1988). A solitary microtransducer is, however, not considered suitable for station pull through anal manometry because they are prone to damage and several readings need to be taken at each station because of the radial variation in pressure (Miller *et al.*, 1988).

The development of the microtransducer recording devices has allowed the extension of the study of the anus and rectum to now include ambulatory studies. Kumar *et al.* (1989) have described a recording system which uses a fine flexible probe on which microtransducers are fixed to measure rectal and anal pressures. This is connected to strain gauge amplifiers and signal encoding circuitry and the data is recorded on magnetic tape on a small data logging cassette recorder.

A portable anorectal manometry unit is now also available for use at the bedside (Orrom *et al.*, 1990).

The reproducibility of anal manometry results has been confirmed in two recent studies (Krogh Pedersen and Christiansen, 1989; Eckhardt and Elmer, 1991).

Recto-anal inhibitory reflex

The recto-anal reflex (Fig. 7) was first described by Gowers (1877) and it has been studied on many occasions since then in humans and animals (Sherrington, 1892; Gaston, 1948; Parks *et al.*, 1962; Schuster *et al.*, 1963; Bennett and Duthie, 1964; Phillips and Edwards, 1965; Kerremans, 1968, 1969; Frenckner and Euler, 1975; Read *et al.*, 1983). The reflex can be elicited by inflating a balloon in the rectum to produce distension. The initial response is a brief contraction of the external sphincter (inflation reflex) which is followed by relaxation of the internal and external sphincters (inhibitory reflex) (Callaghan and Nixon, 1964; Read *et al.*, 1983).

Kerremans (1969) found the threshold volume of rectal distension required to initiate the inhibitory reflex to be between 10 and 30mls.

Read *et al.*, (1983) recorded the reflex by distending a balloon inserted

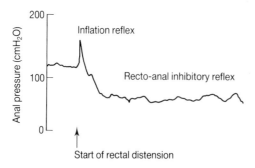

Fig. 7 Normal recto-anal inhibitory reflex in response to rectal distension preceded by external anal sphincter contraction (inflation reflex).

into the rectum with 10ml increments of air whilst measuring anal sphincter pressure. They recorded the volume of distension required to completely inhibit anal sphincter tone for more than 60 seconds. They found the mean volume required in normal subjects to be 77mls.

Electromyography

Electromyography (EMG) (Fig. 8) provides an assessment of the electrical activity generated within the muscle being sampled. The use of an integrated recording system provides information about the amplitude and frequency of the recorded potentials.

The main electromyographic technique used to examine the external anal sphincter and puborectalis muscles has employed the use of concentric EMG needles (Bartolo *et al.*, 1983).

This technique in clinical practice has allowed mapping of external sphincter defects to be performed before surgical repair is attempted and has also been used in research studies of patients with other anorectal abnormalities. The examination, however, does tend to be painful and requires the availability of expensive equipment.

Fine EMG wire electrodes have also been used. These tend to be less painful and can be left in situ during dynamic assessment especially during defaecation (Bartolo *et al.*, 1986).

Surface EMG measurements using either an intra-anal plug (Pinho *et al.*, 1991) or surface electrodes applied to the perianal skin (Kumar *et al.*, 1990) now offer non-invasive methods of recording EMG activity.

Kumar *et al.*, (1990) have described a method of recording 24 hour ambulatory anal EMG and manometry which has lead to improved understanding of normal anorectal physiology.

Other EMG methods and nerve conduction studies can be performed. These are described later (see pages 41–42)

EMG

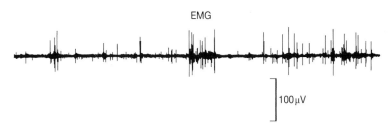

100 µV

Fig. 8 Normal electromyography (EMG) recordings from the external anal sphincter. (Reproduced from Kumar *et al.*, *Dig Dis Sci*; 1990, **35**: 646).

References

Bartolo DCC, Jarratt JA, Read NW. (1983) The use of conventional electromyography to assess external sphincter neuropathy in man. *J Neurol Neurosurg Psychiat*; **46**: 1115–18.
Bartolo DCC, Roe AM, Locke-Edmunds JC, Virjee J, Mortensen NJMcC. (1986) Flap valve theory of anorectal continence. *Br J Surg*. **73**: 1012–1014.

Bennett RC, Duthie HL. (1964) The functional importance of the internal anal sphincter. *Br J Surg;* **51**: 355–7.

Callaghan RP, Nixon HH. (1964) Megarectum: physiological observations. *Arch Dis Childhood;* **39**: 153–7.

Collins CD, Brown BH, Whittaker GE, Duthie HL. (1969). New method of measuring forces in the anal canal. *Gut;* **10**: 160–3.

Collins CD, Duthie HL, Shelley T, Whittaker GE. (1967) Forces in the anal canal and anal continence. *Gut;* **8**: 354–60.

Dickinson VA. (1978) Maintenance of anal continence: a review of pelvic floor physiology. *Gut;* **19**: 1163–1174.

Eckhardt VF, Elmer T. (1991) Reliability of anal pressure measurements. *Dis Colon Rectum;* **34**: 72–77.

Frenckner B, Euler CV. (1975) Influence of pudendal nerve block on the function of the anal sphincters. *Gut;* **16**: 482–489.

Gaston EA. (1948) The physiology of faecal incontinence. *Surg Gynecol Obstet;* **87**: 280–290.

Gowers WR. (1877) The automatic action of the sphincter ani. *Proc Roy Soc;* **26**: 77–84.

Hancock BD. (1976) Measurement of anal pressure and motility. *Gut;* **17**: 645–51.

Henry MM, Parks AG. (1980) The investigation of anorectal function. *Hospital Update;* **6**: 29–41.

Hill JR, Kelley MLJnr, Schlegel JF, Code CF. (1960). Pressure profile of the rectum and anus of healthy persons. *Dis Colon Rectum;* **2**: 203–9.

Kerremans R. (1968) Electrical activity and motility of the internal anal sphincter. *Acta Gastroenterol Belg;* **31**: 465–82.

Kerremans R. (1969) *Morphological and Physiological Aspects of Anal Continence and Defaecation.* Editions Arsica, Brussels.

Krogh Pedersen I, Christiansen J. (1989) A study of the physiological variation in anal manometry. *Br J Surg;* **76**: 69–71.

Kumar D, Waldron D, Williams NS, Browning C, Hutton MRE, Wingate DL. (1990) Prolonged anorectal manometry and external anal sphincter electromyography in ambulant human subjects. *Dis Colon Rectum;* **35**: 641–8.

Kumar D, Williams NS, Waldron D, Wingate DL. (1989) Prolonged manometric recording of anorectal motor activity in ambulant human subjects: evidence of periodic activity. *Gut;* **30**: 1007–11.

McHugh SM, Diamant NE. (1987) Effect of age, gender, and parity on anal canal pressures. *Dig Dis Sci;* **32**: 726–36.

Miller R, Bartolo DCC, James D, Mortensen NJMcC. (1989) Air filled microballoon manometry for use in anorectal physiology. *Br J Surg;* **76**: 72–75.

Miller R, Bartolo DCC, Roe AM, Mortensen NJMcC. (1988) Air filled microballoon manometry for use in anorectal physiology. *Br J Surg;* **75**: 40–43.

Orrom WJ, Williams JG, Rothenberger DA, Wong WD. (1990) Portable anorectal manometry. *Br J Surg;* **77**: 876–7.

Parks AG. Porter NH, Melzak J. (1962) Experimental studies of the reflex mechanism controlling the muscles of the pelvic floor. *Dis Colon Rectum;* **5**: 407–14.

Phillips SF, Edwards DAW. (1965) Some aspects of anal continence and defaecation. *Gut;* **6**: 396–406.

Pinho M, Hosie K, Bielecki K, Keighley MRB. (1991) Assessment of noninvasive intra-anal electromyography to evaluate sphincter function. *Dis Colon Rectum;* **34**: 69–71.

Read NW, Haynes WG, Bartolo DCC et al. (1983) Use of anorectal manometry during rectal infusion of saline to investigate sphincter function in incontinent patients. *Gastroenterology;* **85**: 105–113.

Schuster MM, Hendrix TR, Mendeloff AI. (1963) The internal anal sphincter response: manometric studies on its normal physiology, neural pathways and alteration in bowel disorders. *J Clin Invest*; **42**: 196–207.

Sherrington CS. (1892) Notes on the arrangement of some motor fibres in the lumbo-sacral plexus. Section III motor roots to muscles of the anus. J Physiol; **13**: 621–772.

Wankling WJ, Brown BH, Collins CD, Duthie HL. (1968). Basic electrical activity in the anal canal in man. *Gut*; **9**: 459–60.

4

Maintenance of anal continence

The mechanisms which help to maintain continence are discussed in this chapter.

Anal sphincter pressure zone

The anal sphincters contribute to the maintenance of continence by exerting a higher pressure in the anal canal than in the rectum (Hill et al., 1960; Duthie and Bennett, 1963). This is generated mainly by the internal anal sphincter (Duthie and Watts, 1965; Frenckner and Euler, 1975; Schweiger, 1979) in which continuous electrical activity is present at rest (Kerremans, 1969; Ustach et al., 1970; Wankling et al., 1968). Frenckner and Euler (1975) demonstrated that the internal sphincter contributes approximately 85% of resting anal canal pressure and is 'of major importance for continence at rest'. The operation of internal sphincterotomy is followed by faecal soiling in up to 40% of cases (Bennett and Goligher, 1962; Bennett and Duthie, 1964; Hardy, 1967, 1972; Hoffman and Goligher, 1970).

The external anal sphincter and puborectalis also demonstrate continuous activity (Floyd and Walls, 1953; Taverner and Smiddy, 1959; Porter, 1962; Parks et al., 1962; Melzak and Porter, 1964; Duthie and Watts, 1965; Parks et al., 1966; Kerremans, 1969; Frenckner and Euler, 1975) which is maintained as part of a spinal reflex arc. The reflex arc remains intact in patients with complete transection of the spinal cord in whom tonic activity is present (although slightly modified) (Porter, 1962; Melzak and Porter 1964; Frenckner and Euler, 1975). Tonic activity, however, is lost in patients with tabes dorsalis indicating that sensory input from the pelvic floor is required to maintain the reflex (Melzak and Porter, 1964).

Anal pressures tend to be higher in males and the sphincter is also longer than in females (Sun and Read, 1989). Until recently knowledge about the motility of the anus and rectum was based on short laboratory recordings. Longer laboratory recordings have demonstrated that the internal sphincter exhibits slow wave and ultra slow wave activity (Fig. 9) (Krogh Pedersen and Christiansen, 1989; Sun and Read, 1989). The internal sphincter is also thought to have an antiperistaltic action as a gradient in the frequency of pressure waves has been recorded in the anal canal (Kerremans, 1969; Hancock, 1976; Read, 1983).

Prolonged recordings in ambulatory subjects are now possible (Kumar *et al.*, 1989). This has lead to better understanding of anorectal physiology and supplements the information that is available about upper gastrointestinal motility in which migrating motor complexes (MMC) are well recognised and are easier to study. The MMC has three phases (Fig. 10):

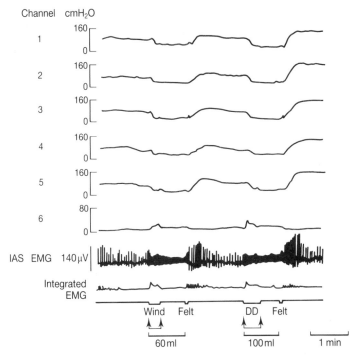

Fig. 9 Recordings of anorectal pressure at ports situated 0·5 to 4·5cm from the anal margin (channels 1 to 6) and the electrical activity of the sphincter complex during distension of a rectal balloon with 60 and 100mls of air. Rectal distension induced, a relaxation in sphincter pressure associated with abolition of the internal anal sphincter (IAS) slow waveactivity and an increase in the activity of the extreme anal sphincter (EAS). Deflation of the balloon produced a rebound increase in pressurewhich is associated with an increase in the amplitude of the IAS slow wave oscillation and a transient increase in EAS electrical activity. DD = desire to defaecate. (Reproduced by permission of the publishers, Butterworth–Heinemann Ltd. from Sun *et al.*, *Int J Colorect Dis*; 1990, **35**: 646)

I.   Quiescence;
II   Irregular contractions;
III Bursts of regular contractions with antegrade propagation.

Kumar *et al.* (1989) have shown clusters of sustained regular rectal activity occuring with a periodicity of 92 minutes. (Fig. 11). This activity resembles phase III activity in the small intestine but lacks the preceding phase of irregular contractions (phase II). It is unclear, however, whether this activity is a continuation of the periodic activity from the upper gastrointestinal tract. The anal canal exhibits bursts of activity in 24 hour recordings but these do not exhibit any evidence of periodic activity.

Kumar *et al.* (1990) found that there is significantly more anal sphincter activity during the day than during the night. External sphincter activity is absent during sleep apart from occasional bursts of activity. Independent bursts of IAS activity occur during sleep.

Anal canal pressure increases during micturition due to an increase in external sphincter activity (Kumar *et al.*, 1990).

Standing or sitting causes a fourfold increase in intrarectal pressure. This is associated with an increase in anal resting pressure (Johnson *et al.*, 1990).

Anal pressure profiles in which anal pressure has been measured at

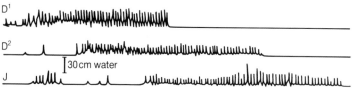

Fig. 10 Normal migrating motor complex recorded from the small intestine. D1 and D2 are recorded from the duodenum and J from the jejunum

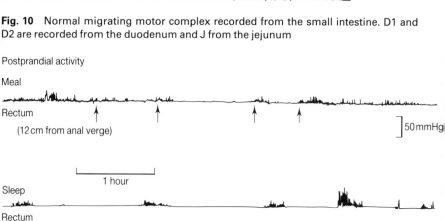

Fig. 11 Continuous record from the rectum of a healthy subject. The top trace shows the effect of a meal on rectal motility. Note the clusters of contractions indicated by the arrows in the postprandial period. The lower trace shows rectal motor complexes during sleep. (Reproduced from Kumar *et al.*, *Gut*; 1989, **30**: 1008)

a number of points within the anal canal demonstrate that the pressure within the canal is not symmetrical. The resting and squeeze pressures are both highest in the outermost part of the anus (Sun and Read, 1989) which suggests that the external sphincter principally surrounds the outermost part of the anal canal (Bannister *et al.*, 1989).

Reflex activity

Tonic activity of the external sphincter makes little contribution to the maintenance of continence (Dickinson, 1978). A maximal voluntary contraction of the external anal sphincter can be maintained for less than one minute (Gaston, 1948; Parks *et al.*, 1962; Duthie and Bennett 1963; Schuster *et al.*, 1965; Philips and Edwards, 1965; Kerremans, 1969) and thus can only serve as an emergency measure to prevent the entry of material into the anal canal. The major contributions of the external sphincter to continence are its reflex activity and voluntary contraction of the sphincter in response to sudden increases in intra-abdominal and rectal pressure.

The effect of rectal distension on the anal sphincters has been extensively investigated by inflating a balloon in the rectum whilst recording pressure in the anal canal. The initial response in the anal sphincter is an increase in pressure (Kerremans, 1969; Frenckner and Euler, 1975; Frenckner, 1975; Varma and Stephens, 1972; Read *et al.*, 1985) which is accompanied by increased electromyographic (EMG) activity in the external anal sphincter which usually lasts for a few seconds (Melzak and Porter, 1964).

This rise in anal pressure, the inflation reflex, is abolished by bilateral pudendal nerve blockade. Frenckner and Euler (1975) calculated that reflex contraction of the external sphincter contributes 60% of the anal canal closing pressure after sudden rectal distension.

Bannister *et al.* (1989) and Sun and Read (1989) have measured anal pressure simultaneously at a number of sites before and during rectal distension in normal subjects. Rectal distension causes a transient increase in anal pressure particularly in the outermost part of the anus due to external sphincter contraction followed by a symmetrical reduction in anal pressure. The electrical activity in the external sphincter, however, increases in amplitude with the degree of distension which suggests that, as the internal sphincter relaxes, the external sphincter contracts in this setting.

The internal sphincter relaxtion and shortening of the anal canal may allow sampling to occur.

Transient increases in intra-abdominal pressure, e.g. during coughing, lead to an increase in external sphincter and puborectalis EMG activity associated with a rise in pressure in the anal canal (Phillips and Edwards, 1965; Kerremans, 1969; Porter, 1962). This is also seen when there is a more prolonged rise in intra-abdominal pressure such as during a Valsalva manoeuvre or straight leg raising (Phillips and Edwards, 1965; Collins *et al.*, 1967; Bartolo *et al.*, 1986). Increasing intra-abdominal pressure by blowing up a balloon causes a similar increase in anal pressure produced by external sphincter activity (Sun and Read, 1989).

Puborectalis muscle and the anorectal angle

The puborectalis muscle plays an important role in the maintenance of continence. Its main action is to maintain an angle between the rectum and the upper anal canal – the anorectal angle (Fig. 3) (Symington, 1888; Kerremans, 1969). This normally has a range of 60–105° (Hardcastle and Parks 1970). Continence is lost when the angle is more obtuse (Kerremans, 1969; Reeve, 1981). Rectal contents are not able to reach the anus when this angle is less than 110°.

Parks *et al.* (1966) suggested that the anorectal angle maintains continence by a flap valve mechanism in which the anterior rectal wall is driven down into the upper anal canal thereby occluding it, with the sphincters subserving fine control. Two recent studies have failed to support this concept (Bartolo *et al.*, 1986; Bannister *et al.*, 1987).

Bartolo *et al.*, (1986) simultaneously measured anal and rectal pressure, and external sphincter and puborectalis muscle EMG activity. They superimposed these recordings on an image intensifier screen displaying the rectum clearly outlined by barium. The anterior rectal wall was always found to be clearly separated from the upper anal canal during a Valsalva manoeuvre in which the intra-abdominal, intrarectal and anal sphincter pressures all increased.

Bannister *et al.* (1987) found in normal subjects that as the pressure within the rectum rose during a Valsalva manoeuvre, the anal pressure was always maintained at a level at least 10cm H_2O higher. Continence clearly was maintained by reflex contraction of the external sphincter. Incontinent patients in contrast were unable to contract the external sphincter sufficiently to keep anal pressure above rectal pressure as intra-abdominal pressure rose. When the test was repeated in these patients after the introduction of 200mls of saline into the rectum, saline leakage occurred whenever rectal pressure exceeded anal pressure.

The flap valve theory appears therefore to have been refuted. Bartolo *et al.* (1986) suggested that the puborectalis muscle acts as a sphincter but Bannister *et al.* (1989) have shown that contraction of the muscle does not alter the pressure in the inner anal canal.

If the anorectal angle is not working via a flap valve mechanism then does it have a role in the preservation of continence? The answer in patients with soft or liquid stools is probably no but in patients with solid or firm stools considerable force would be required to mould stool around an acute angle. The evidence from studies of patients undergoing post anal repair operations which aim to restore continence by recreating the anorectal angle reveal that although they may be successful in restoring continence, this is not necessarily associated with any change in the angle though it does lead to an increase in anal sphincter pressures (Browning and Parks, 1983).

Anorectal sensation and the sampling reflex

The sensory pathways from the anus and rectum are important in the preservation of continence as they give awareness of rectal filling, the need to defaecate and also form the afferent side of a number of complex pelvic floor reflexes. The importance of the reflex and voluntary responses to distension of the rectum has long been recognised. Voluntary contraction of puborectalis and the external sphincter in response to the urge to defaecate is an important temporary measure required during rectal contraction or until the rectum adapts to the new volume and intrarectal pressure is reduced (Porter, 1962). Ihre (1974), Todd (1959) and Meunier *et al.* (1976) have stressed the importance of the level of rectal filling at which the urge to defaecate is experienced. It is necessary to have sufficient margin between the level of filling at which there is awareness of rectal content and the level at which both the internal and external sphincters are reflexly inhibited.

Duthie and Bennett (1963) demonstrated that the upper anal canal reflexly opens to allow intrarectal contents to come into contact with the sensory zone of the anal canal. This sampling response consists of an equalisation of the lower rectal and upper anal canal pressures with the lower anal canal pressure usually unchanged and occurs spontaneously in 90% of normal subjects (Miller *et al.*, 1988a). This occurs frequently and is most frequent when awake and following meals (Kumar *et al.*, 1990).

Miller *et al.* (1988b), in a ambulatory study in which they measured rectal and mid anal canal pressures, demonstrated a median of 7 falls of anal pressure per hour (range 1–41) to such an extent that it was equal to or less than rectal pressure. Sixty percent of these were not felt by the subjects (Fig. 12), perhaps because the rectum was empty and no faeces therefore came into contact with the anal mucosa. In addition to these many other falls in anal pressure occurred in which anal pressure did not fall to or below rectal pressure.

Miller *et al.* (1988b) also observed that passage of flatus occurs without any increase in rectal pressure but with a fall in anal pressure usually below rectal pressure (Fig. 13). Kumar *et al.*, (1990), however, did not find the pattern of anal canal activity during the passage of flatus to be consistent.

Miller *et al.*, (1988c), after careful assessment of anal thermal and mechanical sensitivity as well as mucosal electrosensitivity, confirmed that in normal health the anus is sufficiently sensitive to distinguish between flatus and solid stool. It has been suggested that perhaps thermal sensitivity is important for anal continence as combined mechanical and thermal sensitivity are necessary for sensory discrimination between different substances (Vierck *et al.*, 1986).

The conscious appreciation of the temperature of faeces passing from the rectum into the anal canal does not appear likely to be a major factor in the sampling reflex as Rogers *et al.* (1988) found the mean temperature difference between the rectum and the anal canal to be only 0·13°C. This is unlikely to be detectable as Miller *et al.* (1987) found that the lowest temperature change that the anal canal could detect was 0·8°C.

Read and Read (1982) cast doubt on the importance of anal sensation in continence when they failed to impair anal continence by the application of surface anaesthetic agents within the anal canal. It may be that other continence mechanisms compensated for the loss of sensation.

Data from studies of anal sensation in incontinent patients suggests that it does play a role.

Rectal sensation

Rectal sensation is necessary for the desire to defaecate to be detected. It is, however, not thought to play a significant role in the maintenance

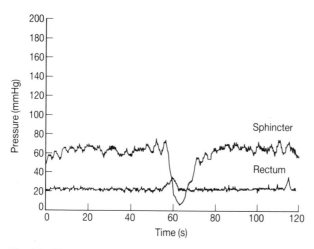

Fig. 12   Simultaneous recording of anal sphincter and rectal pressure which demonstrates the sampling reflex (spontaneous fall in anal pressure below rectal pressure) which was not felt by this normal subject. (Reproduced from Miller *et al.*, *Br J Surg*; 1988, **75**: 1004)

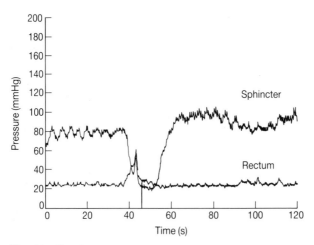

Fig. 13   Simultaneous recording of anal sphincter and rectal pressure on passing flatus. The main change is a fall in anal pressure with a rise in rectal pressure. (Reproduced by permission of the publishers, Butterworth–Heinemann Ltd. from Miller *et al.*, *Br J Surg*; 1988, **75**: 1005)

of continence (see p. 48). In the laboratory it is assessed by balloon distension of the rectum.

Sun *et al.* (1990) in their study found that all their normal subjects perceived rectal sensation within one second of rapid balloon distension of the rectum with 20mls of air. This sensation coincided with contraction of the external anal sphincter and a rectal contraction. Inflation of a rectal balloon with more than 20mls produced a reduction in anal pressure throughout its entire length while 60–70mls of distension induced the greatest reduction of anal pressure. Sustained anal relaxation was not particularly associated with rectal sensation. This study emphasises again the importance of reflex external sphincter contraction in continence maintenance when the rectum is suddenly distended and demonstrates that the anal sphincters can be relaxed without any awareness of rectal distension.

Slit shaped anal canal and mechanical factors

Phillips and Edwards (1965) demonstrated with lateral and anteroposterior radiographs of the rectum and anal canal that the canal is slit shaped and a short segment 0.5 cm long was identified at the junction of the anal canal and rectum which became emptied of barium as the patient moved about. This appeared to correspond to the level of the pelvic diaphragm.

Phillips and Edwards (1965) suggested that the anal canal acts as a flutter valve with intra-abdominal pressure being transmitted, at the level of the levator ani, laterally to the side of the anal canal in the region of the anorectal junction. Duthie (1971), however thought that this was unlikely as no localised zone of increased pressure was identified and puborectalis activity at this level could not be excluded. A flutter valve action was thought unlikely to provide protection against a rise in intrarectal pressure.

Vascular and mucosal component

Longitudinal striations within the anal canal formed by the anal mucosa were demonstrated by Kerremans (1969) who suggested that they may contribute to the complete sealing of the anal canal, probably with some additional effect from the haemorrhoidal sinuses.

The existence of a fluid component from the haemorrhoidal plexus was proposed by Stelzner (1963). This hypothesis has recently been re-examined by Gibbons *et al.* (1986). They fitted measurements of anal sphincter tension and diameter into a mathematical model. Their results suggested that closure of the anal canal was achieved by more than just sphincter contraction.

The anal lining is thick and folded and forms anal cushions (Thomson, 1975; Haas *et al.*, 1984) which are highly vascular spaces that interdigitate to plug the anus at rest. Gibbons *et al.* (1986) proposed that at low sphincter pressures they would tend to swell whereas at higher pressures they would be compressed. When the anal sphincter relaxes this mechanism could maintain closure of the anus by expanding to fill the lumen, and could make an important contribution to the anal resting pressure.

It may account for the observation that patients with hypertrophied anal cushions frequently have higher anal pressures than normal subjects (Hancock and Smith, 1975; Arabi *et al.*, 1977) and that haemorrhoidectomy (which removes a proportion but not all of the vascular tissue in the anal cushion) is often associated with minor degrees of incontinence (Bennett *et al.*, 1963).

References

Arabi Y, Alexander-Williams J, Keighley MRB. (1977) Anal pressure in haemorrhoids and anal fissure. *Am J Surg*; **134**: 608–10.

Bannister JJ, Gibbons C, Read NW. (1987) Preservation of faecal continence during rises in intra-abdominal pressure; is there a role for the flap valve? Gut; **28**: 1242–45.

Bannister JJ, Read NW, Donnelly TC, Sun WM. (1989) External and internal anal sphincter responses to rectal distension in normal subjects and in patients with idiopathic faecal incontinence. *Br J Surg*. **76**: 617–21.

Bartolo DCC, Roe AM, Locke-Edmunds JC, Virjee J, Mortensen NJMcC. (1986) Flap valve theory of anorectal continence. *Br J Surg*; **73**: 1012–1014.

Bennett RC, Duthie HL. (1964) The functional importance of the internal anal sphincter. *Br J Surg*; **51**: 355–7.

Bennett RC, Friedman MHW, Goligher JC. (1963), Late results of haemorrhoidectomy by ligature and excision. *Br Med J*; **2**: 216–219.

Bennett RC, Goligher JC. (1962) Results of internal sphincterotomy for anal fissure. *Br M J*; **2**: 1500–3.

Browning GGP, Parks AG. (1983) Post anal repair for neuropathic faecal incontiennce: correlation of clinical results and anal canal pressures. *Br J Surg*; **70**: 101–4.

Collins CD, Duthie HL, Shelley T, Whittaker GE. (1967) Forces in the anal canal and anal continence. *Gut*; **8**: 354–60.

Dickinson VA. (1978) Maintenance of anal continence: a review of pelvic floor physiology. *Gut*; **19**: 1163–74.

Duthie HL, Bennett RC. (1963) The relation of sensation in the anal canal to the functional anal sphincter; a possible factor in anal continence. *Gut*; **4**: 179–82.

Duthie HL, Watts JM. (1965) Contribution of the external anal sphincter to the pressure zone in the anal canal. *Gut*; **6**: 64–68.

Duthie HL. (1971) Anal continence. *Gut*; **12**: 844–52.

Floyd WF, Walls EW. (1953) Electromyography of the sphincter ani externus in man. *J Physiol*; **122**: 599–609.

Frenckner B. (1975) Function of the anal sphincters in spinal man. *Gut*; **16**: 638–44.

Frenckner B, Euler CV. (1975) Influence of pudendal nerve block on the function of the anal sphincters. *Gut*; **16**: 482–9.

Gaston EA. (1948) The physiology of faecal incontinence. *Surg Gynecol Obstet*; **87**: 280–90.

Gibbons CP, Trowbridge EA, Bannister JJ, Read NW. (1986) Role of anal cushions in maintaining continence. *Lancet*; **i**: 886–8.

Haas PA, Fox TA, Haas GP. (1984) The pathogenesis of haemorrhoids. *Dis Colon Rectum*; **27**: 442–50.

Hancock BD. (1976) Measurement of anal pressure and mobility. *Gut*; **17**: 645–651

Hancock BD, Smith K. (1975) The internal anal sphincter and Lord's procedure for haemorrhoids. *Br J Surg*; **62**: 833–6.

Hardcastle JD, Parks AG. (1970) A study of anal incontinence and some principles of surgical treatment. *Proc Roy Soc Med*; **63**: 116–8.

Hardy KJ. (1967) Internal sphincterotomy. An appraisal with special reference to sequelae. *Br J Surg*; **54**: 30–31.

Hardy K.J. (1972) Involuntary sphincter tone in the maintenance of continence. *Aust NZ J Surg*; **42**: 48–50.

Hill JR, Kelley MLJnr, Schlegel JF, Code CF. (1960) Pressure profile of the rectum and anus of healthy persons. *Dis Colon Rectum*; **2**: 203–9.

Hoffman DC, Goligher JC. (1970) Lateral subcutaneous sphincterotomy in treatment of anal fissure. *Br Med J*; **3**: 673–5.

Ihre T. (1974) Studies on anal function in continent and incontinent patients. *Scand J Gastroentero*; **9**: (Suppl): 25.

Johnson GP, Pemberton JH, Ness J, Samson M, Zinsmeister AR. (1990) Transducer manometry and the effect of body position on anal canal pressures. *Dis Colon Rectum*; **33**: 469–75.

Kerremans R. (1969) *Morphological and Physiological Aspects of Anal Continence and Defaecation*. Editions Arsica, Brussels.

Krogh Pedersen I, Christiansen J. (1989) A study of the physiological variation in anal manometry. *Br J Surg*; **76**: 69–71.

Kumar D, Williams NS, Waldron D, Wingate DL. (1989) Prolonged manometric recording of anorectal motor activity in ambulant human subjects: evidence of periodic activity. *Gut*; **30**: 1007–11.

Kumar D, Waldron D, Williams NS, Browning C, Hutton MRE, Wingate DL. (1990) Prolonged anorectal manometry and external anal sphincter electromyography in ambulant human subjects. *Dis Colon Rectum*; **35**: 641–648.

Melzak J, Porter NH. (1964) Studies of the reflex activity of the external anal sphincter in spinal man. *Paraplegia*; **1**: 277–96.

Meunier P, Mollard P, Marechal JM. (1976) Physiopathology of megarectum: the association of megarectum and encopresis. *Gut*; **17**: 224–7.

Miller R, Bartolo DCC, Cervero F, Mortensen NJMcC. (1987) Anorectal temperature sensation: a comparison of normal and incontinent patients. *Br J Surg*; **74**: 511–15.

Miller R, Bartolo DCC, Cervero F, Mortensen NJMcC. (1988a) Anorectal sampling: a comparison of normal and incontinent patients. *Br J Surg*; **75**: 44–7.

Miller R, Lewis GT, Bartolo DCC, Cervero F, Mortensen NJMcC. (1988b) Sensory discrimination and dynamic activity in the anorectum: evidence using a new ambulatory technique. *Br J Surg*; **75**: 1003–7.

Miller R, Bartolo DCC, Roe A, Cervero F, Mortensen NJMcC. (1988c) Anal sensation and the continence mechanism. *Dis Colon Rectum*; **31**: 433–8.

Parks AG, Porter NH, Hardcastle J. (1966) The syndrome of the descending perineum. *Proc Roy Soc Med*; **59**: 477–82.

Parks AG. Porter NH, Melzak J. (1962) Experimental studies of the reflex mechanism controlling the muscles of the pelvic floor. *Dis Colon Rectum*; **5**: 407–14.

Phillips SF, Edwards DAW. (1965) Some aspects of anal continence and defaecation. *Gut*; **6**: 396–406.

Porter NH. (1962) A physiological study of the pelvic floor in rectal prolapse. *Ann Roy Coll Surg Eng*; **31**: 379–404.

Read MG, Read NW. (1982) Role of anorectal sensation in preserving continence. *Gut*; **23**: 345–7.

Read NW, Haynes WG, Bartolo DCC *etal*. AG. (1983) Use of anorectal manometry during rectal infusion of saline to investigate sphincter function in incontinent patients. *Gastroenterology*; **85**: 105–13.

Read NW, Abouzekry L, Read MG, Howell P, Ottewell D, Donnelly TC. (1985) Anorectal function in elderly patients with faecal impaction. *Gastroenterology*; **89**: 959–66.

Reeve DRE. (1981) Anatomy of the sphincters of the alimentary canal. in Thomas PA, Mann CB, (eds) *Alimentary Sphincters and Their Disorders, pp. 1–26. Macmillan, London.*

Rogers J, Hayward MP, Henry MM, Misiewicz JJ. (1988) Temperature gradient between the rectum and the anal canal: evidence against the role of temperature sensation as a sensory modality in the anal canal of normal subjects. *Br J Surg*; **75**: 1083–5.

Schuster MM, Hookman P, Hendrix TR, Mendeloff AI. (1965) Simultaneous manometric recording of the internal and external anal sphincter reflexes. *Bull Johns Hopkins Hosp*; **116**: 79–88.

Schweiger M. (1979) Method for determining individual contributions of voluntary and involuntry anal sphincters to resting tone. *Dis Colon Rectum*; **22**: 415–16.

Stelzner F. (1963) Die Hamorrhoiden und andere Krankheiten des Corpus Cavernosum Recti und des Analkanals. *Deutsche Medizinische Wochenschrift*; **88**: 689, cited in Brocklehurst JC. (1984) The problem of faecal incontinence. In Hellemans J, Vantrappen G (eds) *Gastro-intestinal Tract Disorders in the Elderly.* Churchill Livingstone, Edinburgh.

Sun WM, Read NW. (1989) Anorectal function in normal human subjects: effect of gender. *Int J Colorect Dis*; **4**: 188–96.

Sun WM, Read NW, Miner PB. (1990) Relation between rectal sensation and anal function in normal subjects and patients with faecal incontinence. *Gut*; **31**: 1056–61.

Symington J. (1888) The rectum and anus. *J Anat Physiol*; **23**: 106–15.

Taverner D, Smiddy FG. (1959) An electromyographic study of the normal function of the external anal sphincter and pelvic diaphragm. *Dis Colon Rectum*; **2**: 153–160.

Thomson WHF. (1975) The nature of haemorrhoids. *Br J Surg*; **62**: 542–52.

Todd IP. (1959) Discussion on rectal incontinence. *Proc Roy Soc Med*; **52**: 91–3.

Ustach TJ, Tobon F, Hambrecht T, Bass DD, Schuster MM. (1970) Electrophysiological aspects of human sphincter function. *J Clin Invest*; **49**: 41–48.

Varma KK, Stephens D. (1972) Neuromuscular reflex of rectal continence. *Aust NZ J Surg.* **41**: 252–63.

Vierck CJ, Greenspan JD, Ritz LA, Yeomans DC. (1986) The spinal pathways contributing to the ascending conduction and descending modulation of pain sensation and reactions. In Yaksh TL (ed) *Spinal Afferent Processing*, pp. 275–329. Plenum Press, New York.

Wankling WJ, Brown BH, Collins CD, Duthie HL. (1968) Basic electrical activity in the anal canal in man. *Gut.* **9**: 459–60.

5

Normal defaecation

The act of defaecation is initiated by the movement of faeces from the colon into the rectum. Normal defaecation is therefore dependent upon the normal transit of material through the gut from mouth to anus.

Gut transit

Whole gut transit has been assessed using many different techniques. These methods have been reviewed by Truelove (1966) and have included the ingestion of dyes, millet seed and glass beads. Ritchie (1968) demonstrated that in constipated individuals barium taken by mouth takes longer to reach the rectum than in normal subjects or patients with diarrhoea.

More recently, radio-opaque markers have been used to assess whole gut transit. The transit has been measured by either regular abdominal radiographs or a collection of the patient's stool. Hinton *et al.* (1969) used the latter method to investigate 25 normal male subjects and found that they had all passed the first marker by the end of the third day and all but one had passed 80% of the markers by the end of the fifth day, which they regarded as the upper limit of normal. No subject had passed all the markers by the end of the first day.

These results are consistent with those of workers using other methods (Cummings *et al.*, 1976) but apply only to a Euro-American culture since transit time appears to be related to the amount of dietary fibre. Shorter transit times are reported in populations taking a high fibre diet than in populations taking a refined diet (Burkitt *et al.*, 1972).

Colonic Activity

The movement of faeces from the colon into the rectum occurs as a result of a series of mass movements. The term gastrocolic reflex has frequently been used to describe these mass movements but they are neither gastric nor reflex in origin (Christensen, 1981). It is also clear that central connections are not essential for defaecation as it still occurs in patients with spinal cord transection.

The main stimuli for mass movements are physical activity and the ingestion of food (Holdstock *et al.*, 1970; Holdstock and Misiewicz, 1970; Duthie, 1978). Holdstock and Misiewicz (1970) found that colonic motility increased during and after a meal and that this was associated with propulsive activity in physically active subjects but not in resting subjects (Holdstock *et al.*, 1970). Rectosigmoid motility has also been found to increase after a meal (Roe *et al.*, 1986). The postprandial increase in colonic activity is similar in patients with total gastrectomy, pernicious anaemia and duodenal ulcer which suggests that it is not dependent upon the presence of the stomach, gastric acid, antral gastrin or vagal innnervation (Holdstock and Misiewicz, 1970).

The colonic transit associated with this activity does not appear to be influenced by physical training in normal subjects (Bingham and Cummings, 1989). Their study subjects were 14 young people with a sedentary lifestyle. During the control period, however, they were still 'active' i.e. walking for up to 15 minutes per day, which is probably sufficient physical activity to stimulate colonic motility.

Oettle (1991), however, found that moderate exercise (jogging or cycling) for one hour every day was associated with significantly shorter whole gut tansit times. In the control period of normal activity mean whole gut tansit time was 51·2 hours (95% confidence intervals 41·9–60·5) compared with 36·6 hours (31·6–39·2) for cycling and 34·0 hours (28·8–39·2) for the jogging period.

Kamm *et al.*, (1988) have developed the technique of dynamic colonic scintigraphy to assess colonic motor function. The technique requires the peroral intubation of the right colon using the method described by Kerlin *et al.* (1983). This involves the use of a fine polyvinyl chloride (PVC) tube with a mercury weighted capsule at the tip surrounded by an inflatable balloon. This is swallowed and passes through the small bowel into the colon.

On the morning of the test, subjects are fasted and placed under a large field view gamma camera which encompasses the entire colon and rectum. A radio-isotope 99m Tc-DTPA is then infused into the colon through the tube followed a few minutes later by a dose of bisacodyl to stimulate colonic activity. In normal subjects the radio-isotope moves rapidly from the right colon into the rectum (mean 5·3 minutes) (Fig. 14).

Krevsky *et al.* (1986) used a similar method to assess normal individuals but they did not administer bisacodyl. They followed the progression of the radio-isotope from the caecum to the toilet over a period of 48 hours. They found that the caecum and ascending colon empty rapidly with a

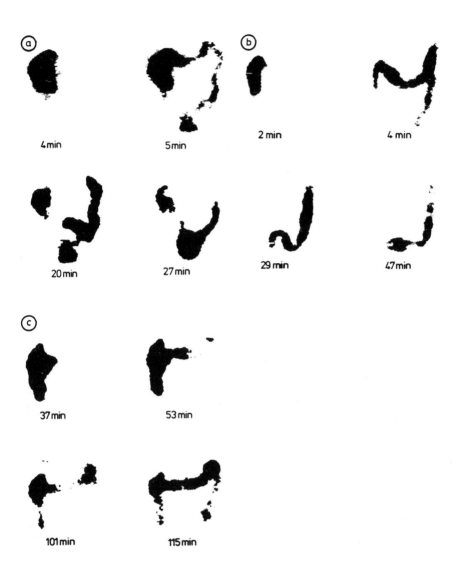

Fig. 14 Three dynamic colonic scintigraphy scans which demonstrate therange of abnormalities. The positions of the 'isotope head' at different times as well as the position of the bulk of the mass of radioactivity can be clearly seen. The time beneath each frame refers to the time from infusion of bisacodyl. (a) A normal subject. Two successive one-minute frames (4 and 5 minutes) show transport of isotope from the hepatic flexure to the rectum in one minute. Most of the isotope has reached the rectum by 27 minutes. (b) Patient with rapid movement to the descending colon, but delayed movement through the sigmoid and rectum. (c) Patient who showed very slow transit throughout the entire colon. Isotope had still not reached the rectum after two hours. (reproduced from Kamm *et al*; *Gut* 1988 29: 1088)

mean half-emptying time of 88 minutes. The transverse colon appears to be the main site for faecal storage.

Reddy *et al.* (1991) have described a technique of simultaneously measuring colonic pressure using a catheter introduced into the transverse colon using a colonoscope and transit of intraluminal colonic contents using the same catheter to introduce the isotope for scintigraphy. They found that intraluminal pressure increased after a meal and that this was greater in the descending colon than in other regions of the colon. Transit was quiescent during fasting; eating stimulated both antegrade and retrograde transit. Postprandial propagating contractions occurred with a mean ($\pm$ SEM) frequency of 0.9 ± 0.3/hour. The corresponding result for ulcerative colitis patients with diarrhoea is $4.5 ° 0.5$/hour.

This functional divide between the left and right colon has also been demonstrated by Waldron *et al.* (1989) who studied patients with transverse colostomies awaiting closure. They found that resistance to balloon distension was greatest in the descending colon. Pooled results from *in vivo* and post mortem studies suggest that there is an active muscular component in the response to distension in the right colon whereas the distal colon has a totally passive response to distension.

Rectal activity

Study of the contractile activity of the rectum was limited to short periods of study until the development of the equipment capable of prolonged ambulatory manometry recordings. Kumar *et al.* (1989) have reported evidence of periodic activity in the rectum. They called these bursts of regular sustained rectal contractions the 'rectal motor complex'. They suggest that these resemble the phase III of the migrating motor complex (MMC) (see Figs. 10 and 11) but in a separate study no evidence could be found that the activity in the small intestine was synchronous with that in the rectum (Kumar *et al.*, 1990).

Prior *et al.* (1991) have performed a further study of anorectal and duodenal motor activity by prolonged nocturnal recordings. They found evidence of runs of regular rectal contractions preceded and followed by motor quiesecence in ten of their 12 normal subjects, which were similar to the 'rectal motor complex' described by Kumar *et al.* (1989). Prior *et al.* doubted the validity of the term rectal motor complex as they found considerable inter-and intrasubject variability with a duration of 3–30 minutes (median 9·0) and periods of 10–420 minutes between the runs of contractile activity. There was no evidence of propagation of this activity through the rectum and the phasic motor activity rarely occurred simultaneously at more than one rectal recording site. There was no consistent relationship with phase III of the small intestinal migrating motor complex. The function of this activity is not clear.

Rectal response to distension

A variety of methods of assessing the rectal motility response to distension have been used over the last few years. Brocklehurst (1951), in his studies of 'senile incontinent' patients, used techniques adapted from

Garry's (1933) studies on cats and Langworthy and Rosenberg's (1939a, 1939b) studies of both cats and humans. Brocklehurst recorded rectal pressure whilst distending a balloon in the rectum with 50ml increments of air. A similar method has more recently been used in a series of studies by Read *et al.* (1983, 1985, Read and Abouzekry (1986) and others (Godec and Cass, 1980; Bubrick *et al.*, 1980).

White *et al.* (1940) attempted the first colonometrogram by filling the entire colon with water. This, however, was a difficult and messy technique which was not accepted in clinical practice.

Preston *et al.* (1983) described a method for performing a proctometrogram in the investigation of severely constipated patients which involved distending a balloon in the rectum with water from a constant infusion pump whilst measuring rectal pressure. The reproducibility of an adaptation of this technique was demonstrated by Varma and Smith (1986). In their system pressure was measured by a microtransducer situated within the balloon though they comment that it can also be measured using a water filled balloon catheter system. The proctometrogram provides information on rectal pressure during rectal distension, rectal motility, rectal compliance and rectal sensation.

The initial response to rectal distension is a rectal contraction (Fig. 15). In many normal subjects regular rectal contractions occur in response to continued distension (Read *et al.*, 1985; Barrett, 1988) (Fig. 16).

During a proctometrogram there is a steady rise in rectal pressure from which rectal compliance can be calculated (Fig. 17). Kendall *et al.* (1990) performed a series of proctometrograms on healthy adult volunteers and found that the pressure-volume responses of the normal rectum to distension are reasonably consistent in individual patients but responses differ widely between individuals. They also found that compliance varies throughout a single rectal trace and between traces which suggests that in any individual, rectal compliance cannot be expressed as a single value. Kendall *et al.* concluded that this technique is not particularly useful in the investigation of rectal function because of the wide range of normality despite Varma and Smith's (1986) initial comments that the technique was reproducible.

Manovolumetry is a new technique in which the rectum is distended at a constant pressure. It has been used to assess rectal function. Akervall *et al* (1989), in a study of normal subjects, found that the rectal response has 3 phases. In the initial phase A, there is rapid rectal distension. Phase B is characterised by a rectal contraction which temporarily reverses or impedes inflow into the rectum. Ninety one percent of the normal subjects studied exhibited regular rectal contractions in this phase but these were abolished by increasing the rectal pressure above 50cm H_2O. In phase C continued rectal distension was found to be associated with very little, if any, rectal activity. This is an ideal property for an organ with a reservoir function. Considerable interindividual variation in rectal compliance was found amongst normal subjects (Akervall *et al.*, 1989).

Akervall *et al.* have also found that a close association exists between the pressure threshold to produce the sensation of rectal filling and the pressure required to elicit the recto-anal inhibitory reflex. They suggest that the anal relaxation that occurs at the onset of rectal sensation is the sampling reflex (see p. 48).

Sun *et al.* (1990) have also found that the sensory and reflex responses to rectal distension vary markedly according to the rate and pattern

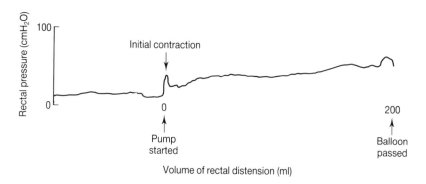

Fig. 15   Proctometrogram demonstrating an initial rectal contraction at the start of rectal distention followed by a slow increase in rectal pressure with rectal distention. The rectal balloon was involuntarily expelled following a rectal contraction.

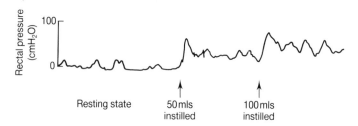

Fig. 16   Rectal pressure recording following rectal distention with 50ml increments of air into a balloon in a normal subject. A single large contraction is seen following the installation of the first 50mls of air. The second 50mls of air provoked large regular rectal contractions.

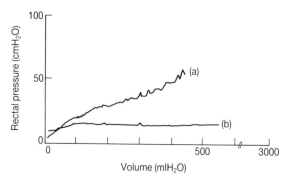

Fig. 17   Proctometrograms from (a) a normal subject and (b) a patient with acquired megacolon.

of rectal distension. The onset of rectal sensation occurred at lower volumes at low infusion rates when the slope of the pressure volume curve was shallower than at high infusion rates. The receptor triggering rectal sensation was therefore not considered a simple volume or pressure receptor but was thought more likely to be due to a slowly adapting mechanoreceptor lying parallel to the circular muscle of the rectal wall. These variations in response may depend upon activation of different populations of mechanoreceptors as well as modulation by rectal motor responses.

Recto-anal inhibitory reflex

The recto-anal inhibitory reflex was first recorded by Gowers (1877) when he measured the anal canal pressure in three patients with faecal incontinence, two of whom were paraplegics. Despite their incontinence and absence of voluntary control, he noted that in each case the sphincter was in a state of continuous contraction and that it could be inhibited by the injection of air into the rectum. Since there was no external sphincter muscle activity in these patients, he concluded that only the internal sphincter was concerned with this reflex, which he also found in normal subjects.

Denny Brown and Robertson (1935) examined the recto-anal reflex further in their investigation of the nervous control of defaecation, and found it to be present in normal subjects, patients with transverse lesions of the cord and patients with sacral root lesions. The reflex was induced by tension in the wall of the rectum. They concluded that it was nervous in mechanism and independent of the central nervous system, since it was present in all of the patients that they studied. They postulated that it was related to the intramural ganglionic plexus. They found that the reflex diminished with increasing distance between the rectal balloon and the internal sphincter.

The reflex response of the internal sphincter to distension is normally present from the sixth day of life (Howard and Nixon, 1968). It is, however absent in patients with Hirschsprung's disease in which intramural ganglia are absent from the rectum and colon (Callaghan and Nixon, 1964; Lawson and Nixon, 1967; Howard and Nixon, 1968; Arhan *et al.*, 1972; Varma and Stephens, 1972; Meunier and Mollard, 1977) which sugests that an intact myenteric plexus is required for the presence of the reflex.

Lubowski *et al.* (1987) have demonstrated that the reflex is not mediated via the sympathetic innervation as it cannot be blocked by bilateral presacral nerve blockade. The reflex is, however, lost following full circumference myotomy of the rectum down to the submucosal layer, suggesting that it is dependent upon the myenteric plexus.

The reflex is also usually absent after proctectomy and colo-anal anastomosis but in some patients it returns after 1–3 years (Lane and Parks, (1977). The return of the reflex suggests that the nerve plexus re-establishes itself across the anastomosis, which is supported by Kiff *et al.*'s (1977) demonstration that the myenteric plexus can cross such an anastomosis.

The act of defaecation

Normal defaecation should follow the mass movement of faeces into the rectum, especially when rectal distension is of sufficient degree to produce the sensation of the desire to void. If it is socially acceptable for defaecation to proceed, a number of events need to occur to enable this, as the continence mechanisms need to be relaxed to allow the expulsion of faeces.

These events have been demonstrated in simulated defaecation studies of normal individuals. Womack *et al.* (1985) performed a defaecating proctography study with simultaneous recording of external sphincter EMG activity. They found that all their normal subjects were able to void contrast media without difficulty. During voiding, intrarectal pressure increased, sphincter activity decreased and the anorectal angle became more obtuse as the pelvic floor descended. The increased anorectal angle is thought to be due to the relaxation of the puborectalis muscle that is known to occur at this stage (Roe *et al.*, 1986; Read *et al.*, 1986; Parks *et al.*, 1966).

Perineal descent on defaecatory straining of up to 3cm below the pubococcygeal line may occur in normal subjects (Roe *et al.*, 1986). More extensive descent is abnormal.

Expulsion of faeces in defaecation requires intrarectal pressure to be higher than anal pressure and to be of sufficient magnitude to push faeces through any residual anorectal angle. This process is usually under some degree of voluntary control.

Intra-abdominal pressure is increased by contraction of the abdominal wall musculature and the diaphragm which causes an increase in intrarectal pressure of 70–100 cmH$_2$O (Lennard-Jones 1985). The extent to which the regular rectal contractions that are induced by rectal distension (Read et al 1986; Akervall *et al.*, 1989) may also help in the expulsion of faeces during defaecation is uncertain.

At the start of defaecatory straining EMG activity in the external sphincter increases and is then followed by complete inhibition of its activity (Parks *et al.*, 1962). Some apparently normal individuals, however, are able to defaecate through sphincters that do not relax (Kerremans, 1969).

At the end of defaecation there is a rapid burst of activity in the external sphincter and pelvic floor muscles to restore tone and the anorectal angle (Porter, 1962) and the pelvic floor is returned to the resting position (Womack *et al.*, 1986). This has been called the closing reflex or post defaecation reflex (Parks *et al.*, 1966).

If the urge to defaecate is resisted, the external anal sphincter contracts, the intrarectal pressure drops and the ano-rectal angle is reestablished. The rectal contents may then either return to the sigmoid colon or remain in the rectum. The presence of faeces in the rectum is not necessarily an abnormal finding (Goligher and Hughes, 1951; Donald *et al.*, 1985).

The quantity of faeces passed at defaecation may vary from the partial contents of the rectum to the whole contents of the rectum and descending colon.

Simulated defaecation studies in normal individuals have revealed that the ability to defaecate is related to the consistency and size of a stool as it takes longer and requires the use of higher intra-abdominal pressures to pass small hard stools than a large soft stool (Bannister *et al.*, 1987). Individuals trying to pass hard pellets would therefore appear to be at greater risk of becoming constipated.

References

Akervall S, Fasth S, Nordgren S, Oresland T, Hulten L. (1989) Rectal reservoir and sensory function studied by graded isobaric distension in normal man. *Gut*; **30**: 496–502.

Arhan P, Faverdin C, Thouvent J. (1972) Anorectal motility in sick children. *Scand J Gastroenterol*; **7**: 309–14.

Bannister JJ, Davison P, Timms JM, Gibbons C, Read NW. (1987) Effect of stool size and consistency on defaecation. *Gut*; **28**: 1246–50.

Barrett JA. (1988) A study of the anorectal pathophysiology of geriatric patients with faecal incontinence. MD thesis. University of Liverpool.

Bingham SA, Cummings JH. (1989) Effect of physical exercise and fitness on large intestinal function. *Gastroenterology*; **97**: 1389–99.

Brocklehurst JC. (1951) *Incontinence in Old Age*. Churchill Livingstone, Edinburgh.

Bubrick MP, Godec CJ, Cass AS. (1980) Functional evaluation of the rectal ampulla with the ampullometrogram. *J Roy Soc Med*; **73**: 234–7.

Burkitt DP, Walker ARP, Painter NS. (1972) Effect of dietary fibre on stools and transit-times, and its role in the causation of disease. *Lancet*; **ii**: 1408–11.

Callaghan RP, Nixon HH. (1964) Megarectum: physiological observations. *Arch Dis Childhood*; **39**: 153–7.

Christensen J. (1981) The controls of gastrointestinal movements: some old and new views. *New Eng J Med*; **285**: 85–98.

Cummings JH, Jenkins DJA, Wiggins HS. (1976) Measurement of the mean transit time of dietary residue through the human gut. *Gut*; **17**: 210–18.

Denny Brown DE, Robertson EG. (1935) An investigation of the nervous control of defaecation. *Brain*; **58**: 256–310.

Donald IP, Smith RG, Cruikshank JG, Elton RA, Stoddart ME. (1985) A study of constipation in the elderly living at home. *Gerontology*; **31**: 112–18.

Duthie HL. (1978) Colonic response to eating. *Gastroenterology*; **75**: 527–9.

Garry RC. (1933) The nervous control of the caudal region of the large bowel in the cat. *J Physiol*; **77**: 422–31.

Godec CJ, Cass AS. (1980) Comparison of pressure measurements in the lower urinary and faecal pathways. *J Urol*; **123**: 58–60.

Goligher JC, Hughes ESR. (1951) Sensibility of the rectum and colon: its role in the mechanism of anal continence. *Lancet*. **i**: 543–8.

Gowers WR. (1877) The automatic action of the sphincter ani. *Proc Roy Soc*; **26**: 77–84.

Hinton JM, Lennard-Jones JE, Young AC. (1969) A new method for studying gut transit times using radioopaque markers. *Gut*; **10**: 842–7.

Holdstock DJ, Misiewicz JJ. (1970) Factors controlling colonic motility: Colonic pressures and transit after meals in patients with total gastrectomy, pernicious anaemia or duodenal ulcer. *Gut*; **11**: 100–10.

Holdstock DJ, Misiewicz JJ, Smith T, Rowlands EN. (1970) Propulsion (mass movements) in the human colon and its relationship to meals and somatic activity. *Gut*; **11**: 91–9.

Howard ER, Nixon HH. (1968) Internal anal sphincter. Observations on development and mechanisms of inhibitory responses in premature infants and children with Hirschsprung's disease. *Arch Dis Childhood*; **43**: 569–78.

Kamm MA, Lennard-Jones JE, Thompson DG, Sobnack R, Garvie NW, Gransowska M. (1988) Dynamic scanning defines a colonic defect in severe idiopathic constipation. *Gut*; **29**: 1085–92.

Kendall GPN, Thompson DG, Day SJ, Lennard-Jones JE. (1990) Inter-and intraindividual variation in pressure-volume relations of the rectum in normal subjects and patients with the irritable bowel syndrome. *Gut*; **31**: 1062–8.

Kerlin P, Tucker R, Phillips SF. (1983) Rapid intubation of the ileocolonic region of man. *Aust NZ J Med*; **13**: 591–593.

Kerremans R. (1969) *Morphological and Physiological Aspects of Anal Continence and Defaecation*. Editions Arsica, Brussels.

Kiff ES, Lord MG, Gosling JA. (1977) A study of intramural autonomic nerves in relation to a large bowel anastomosis in the rat. *J Anat*; **128**: 428–9.

Krevsky B, Malmud LS, D'Ercole F, Maurer AH, Fisher RS. (1986) Colonic transit scintigraphy. A physiologic approach to the quantitative measurement of colonic transit in humans. *Gastroenterology*; **91**: 1102–1112.

Kumar D, Thompson PD, Wingate DL. (1990) Absence of synchrony between human small intestinal migrating motor complex and rectal motor complex. *Am J Physiol*; **258**: G171–2.

Kumar D, Williams NS, Waldron D, Wingate DL. (1989) Prolonged manometric recordings of anorectal motor activity in ambulant human subjects: evidence of periodic activity. *Gut*; **30**: 1007–11.

Lane RHS, Parks AG. (1977) Function of the anal sphincters following colo- anal anastomosis. *Br J Surg*; **64**: 596–599.

Langworthy OR, Rosenberg SJ. (1939a) The control by the central nervous system of the rectal smooth muscle. *J Neurol*; **2**: 356.

Langworthy OR, Rosenberg SJ. (1939b) Abnormalities of rectal tone and contraction in paraplegia and hemiplegia. *Am J Dig Dis*; **6**: 455–8.

Lawson JN, Nixon HH. (1967) Anal canal pressures in the diagnosis of Hirschsprung's disease. *J Paed Surg*; **2**: 544–52.

Lennard-Jones JE. (1985) Pathophysiology of constipation. *Br J Surg*; **72** (Suppl): S7–S8

Lubowski DZ, Nicholls RJ, Swash M, Jordan MJ. (1987) Neural control of internal anal sphincter function. *Br J Surg*; **74**: 668–70.

Meunier P, Mollard P. (1977) Control of the internal anal sphincter (manometric study with human subjects). *Pflugers Archiv*; **370**: 233–9.

Oettle GJ. (1991) Effect of moderate exercise on bowel habit. *Gut*; **32**: 941–4.

Parks AG, Porter NH, Hardcastle J. (1966) The syndrome of the descending perineum. *Proc Roy Soc Med*; **59**: 477–82.

Parks AG. Porter NH, Melzak J. (1962) Experimental studies of the reflex mechanism controlling the muscles of the pelvic floor. *Dis Colon Rectum*; **5**: 407–14.

Porter NH. (1962) A physiological study of the pelvic floor in rectal prolapse. *Ann Roy Coll Surg Eng*; **31**: 379–404.

Preston DM, Barnes PRH, Lennard-Jones JE. (1983) Proctometrogram: does it have a role in the evaluation of adults with constipation? *Gut*; **24**: A1010–11.

Prior A, Fearn UJ, Read NW. (1991) Intermittent rectal motor activity: a rectal motor complex? *Gut*; **32**: 1360–3.

Read NW, Abouzekry L. (1986) Why do patients with faecal impaction have faecal incontinence? *Gut*; **27**: 283–7.

Read NW, Abouzekry L, Read MG, Howell P, Ottewell D, Donnelly TC. (1985) Anorectal function in elderly patients with faecal impaction. *Gastroenterology*; **89**: 959–66.

Read NW, Haynes WG, Bartolo DCC, *et al.* (1983) Use of anorectal manometry during rectal infusion of saline to investigate sphincter function in incontinent patients. *Gastroenterology*; **85**: 105–13.

Read NW, Timms JM, Barfield LJ, Donnelly TC, Bannister JJ. (1986) Impairment of defaecation in young women with severe constipation. *Gastroenterology*; **90**: 53–60.

Reddy SN, Bazzocchi G, Chan S *et al.* (1991) Colonic motility and transit in health and ulcerative colitis. *Gastroenterology*; **101**: 1289–97.

Ritchie JA. (1968) Colonic motor activity and bowel function. Part II Distribution and incidence of motor activity at rest and after food and carbachol. *Gut*; **9**: 502–11.

Roe AM, Bartolo DCC, Mortensen NJMcC. (1986) Diagnosis and surgical management of intractable constipation. *Br J Surg*; **73**: 854–61.

Sun WM, Read NW, Prior A, Daly JA, Cheah SK, Grundy D. (1990) Sensory and motor responses to rectal distension vary according to rate and pattern of balloon inflation. *Gastroenterology*; **99**: 1008–15.

Truelove SC. (1966) Movement of the large intestine. *Physiol Rev*; **46**: 457–512.

Varma JS, Smith AN. (1986) Reproducibility of the proctometrogram. *Gut*; **27**: 288–92.

Varma KK, Stephens D. (1972) Neuromuscular reflex of rectal continence. *Aust NZ J Surg*; **41**: 252–263.

Waldron DJ, Gill RC, Bowes KL. (1989) Pressure response of human colon to intraluminal distension. *Dig Dis Sci*; **34**: 1163–7.

White JC, Verlot MG, Ehrentheil O. (1940) Neurogenic disturbances of the colon and their investigation by the colonmetrogram. *Ann Surg;*. **112**: 1042–57.

Womack NR, Morrison JFB, Williams NS. (1986) The role of pelvic floor denervation in the aetiology of idiopathic faecal incontinence. *Br J Surg*; **73**: 404–7.

Womack NR, Williams NS, Holmfield JHM, Morrison JFB, Simpkins KC. (1985) New method for the dynamic assessment of anorectal function in constipation. *Br J Surg*; **72**: 994–8.

6

Anorectal incontinence (idiopathic faecal incontinence)

This type of incontinence has been the subject of a great deal of research. The underlying functional disorder in anorectal incontinence is weakness of the anal sphincter and pelvic floor muscles with or without anorectal sensory loss. The term 'anorectal incontinence' is used in preference to 'idiopathic faecal incontinence' as specific causes have now been identified or 'neurogenic faecal incontinence' as this term has been used to describe another type of incontinence.

Direct injury to the anal sphincter

Division of the anal sphincter muscles is recognised as a cause of faecal incontinence. It may occur during surgery or be due to trauma, e.g. sphincter tear during childbirth .

The investigation of defects, particularly in the external anal sphincter, has until recently been performed by using anal manometry and concentric needle electromyography as it is not always possible to detect the defects accurately on digital examination. Anal endosonography is a technique that can now be used to identify defects accurately with minimal discomfort (Law *et al.*, 1990).

Using this technique, Law *et al.*, (1991) found that 85% of patients with incontinence of traumatic origin had external sphincter defects. Thirty nine percent of these patients also have internal sphincter defects which previously had escaped recognition with EMG mapping techniques.

Anal sphincter injury after anal dilation has also been demonstrated using this technique (Speakman *et al.*, 1991).

External anal sphincter and pelvic floor muscle weakness

Manometry studies

Patients with anorectal incontinence, with or without rectal prolapse, have been shown on anorectal manometry to have lower anal resting tone and lower maximal voluntary contraction pressure than comparable controls (Porter, 1962; Read *et al.*, 1979; Henry *et al.*, 1980; Neill *et al.*, 1981; Matheson and Keighley, 1981; Read *et al.*, 1984; Kiff and Swash, 1984a; Snooks *et al.*, 1985b).

Felt Bersma *et al.* (1990) found that the maximal anal squeeze pressure was the most discriminative test predicting continence in patients with anorectal incontinence but continence could not be predicted solely on the basis of the squeeze pressure presumably because of the multifactorial nature of the maintenance of continence.

EMG studies

Conventional EMG studies of incontinent patients have shown that the amplitude of action potentials recorded in the external anal sphincter and puborectalis muscles is reduced both at rest and during maximal voluntary contraction (Neill *et al.*, 1981; Kiff and Swash 1984b).

Histological studies

The observation that the anorectal angle is frequently lost on straining in incontinent patients (Hardcastle and Parks, 1970) lead Parks (1967) to introduce the operation of post-anal repair. The aim of this operation was to restore the anorectal angle and continence in these patients with severe anorectal incontinence. Whilst operating on 25 patients with long standing anorectal incontinence, Parks biopsied the external anal sphincter, puborectalis and levator ani muscles and found histological evidence of denervation which was most marked in the external sphincter muscle (Parks *et al.*, 1977).

Histometric studies in a similar group of patients revealed a marked loss of muscle fibres in the external sphincter which was replaced by fibrous tissue in some patients (Beersiek *et al.*, 1979). The mean diameters of the remaining type 1 and type 2 fibres were increased in all of the specimens studied. Fibre hypertrophy in the external sphincter and puborectalis muscles was accompanied by increased variability in fibre diameter. They considered the multiple peaks on their histogram of fibre diameters to be consistent with partial reinnervation. These changes are consistent with neuropathy as denervation of some muscle fibres may result in compensatory hypertrophy of others (Schwartz *et al.*, 1976, Swash 1980).

Anal reflex

The anal reflex, originally reported by Rossolimo (1891), is absent on clinical examination in many patients with anorectal incontinence (Parks, 1975). A technique of measuring the latency of the anal reflex was developed by Henry and Swash (1978). They supramaximally stimulated the perianal skin and recorded the response in the external sphincter. They found the mean latency of the reflex prolonged from a normal of 8.3 msec to 13.0 msec in 22 incontinent patients (Henry *et al.*, 1980) and concluded that this supported the concept of denervation being the major cause of anorectal incontinence. Neill *et al.* (1981) subsequently demonstrated similar prolongation of the anal reflex latency in patients with faecal incontinence with and without rectal prolapse, but not in patients with rectal prolapse alone.

The validity of the method has however been questioned since the latency of the reflex was much shorter than that of 50 msec recorded by Pedersen *et al.* (1978). However to avoid amplifier saturation these workers had blocked the first 20 msec of their response and therefore missed the early response (Swash, 1982; Pedersen *et al.*, 1982). Early and late components of the reflex were therefore recognised.

The early component was not considered to represent the spinal reflex as the latency for conduction from L1 to the anal verge following direct transcutaneous stimulation of the spinal cord is 7 msec (Marsden *et al.*, 1982; Kiff and Swash, 1984b). Direct spread of the stimulus current to small branches of the pudendal innervation of the external sphincter is thought to account for the early response (Swash, 1982; Pedersen *et al.*, 1982; Vodusek *et al.*, 1983; Bartolo *et al.*, 1983a; Wright *et al.*, 1985).

The late component (latency 30–60 ms) is accepted as representing the spinal reflex but the wide range of latency in normal individuals (Wright *et al.*, 1985) and the lack of correlation with other indices of external sphincter neuropathy (Bartolo *et al.*, 1983a) indicate that the technique is an inadequate means of demonstrating nerve damage in patients with anorectal incontinence.

Single fibre EMG studies

Single fibre electromyography as described by Stalberg and Thiele (1975) is a method used to measure the fibre density within a muscle. Increased fibre density, in a muscle known not to be affected by myopathy, is consistent with re-innervation due to collateral axonal sprouting (Stalberg and Trontelj, 1979).

Neill and Swash (1980) measured the fibre density within the external sphincter in 13 normal subjects and found it to be similar to that found in other striated muscles (Stalberg and Trontelj, 1979). A significant increase in fibre density in both the external sphincter and the puborectalis muscles has been found in patients with anorectal incontinence (Neill *et al.*, 1981b; Snooks *et al.*, 1985). Fibre density is correlated with the severity of incontinence.

Similar evidence of partial denervation with prolongation of motor unit potentials measured during conventional EMG has been found in both the external sphincter and puborectalis muscles in patients with anorectal incontinence (Bartolo *et al.*, 1983b, 1983c). Partial denervation was also noted in both muscles in patients with the descending perineum syndrome and in the external sphincter, but not the puborectalis, in patients with chronic constipation.

Pudendal nerve conduction studies

The innervation of the external anal sphincter is now accessible to study as the pudendal nerves can be stimulated transrectally and the latency to the response in the external sphincter measured (pudendal nerve terminal motor latency). This latency is prolonged in patients with anorectal incontinence (3·1 ms) compared with normal controls (2·0 ms) (Kiff and Swash, 1984a). The pudendal neuropathy may, however, be asymmetrical (Lubowski *et al.*, 1988a).

The proximal innervation can also be assessed and has also been studied by transcutaneous stimulation of nerve roots at the level of the L1 and L4 vertebrae. The latency to the response in the external sphincter is prolonged in patients with anorectal incontinence though the proximal conduction between L1 and L4 is normal (Kiff and Swash, 1984b; Snooks *et al.*, 1985b) suggesting that in these patients the conduction delay to the external sphincter occurs in the distal segment of the pudendal nerve. A conduction delay has also been demonstrated from L1 to the puborectalis muscle (Snooks *et al.*, 1985b).

Denervation of the external anal sphincter and pelvic floor muscles has therefore been demonstrated in patients with anorectal incontinence. A number of possible causes for this have been proposed which include stretch injury of the pudendal or perineal nerves due to pelvic floor descent induced by either direct damage to the nerve during childbirth or chronic straining at stool. Entrapment of the pudendal nerve under the sacrospinous ligament has also been suggested as a possible cause.

Obstetric factors

Most patients presenting to surgical units with ano-rectal incontinence are female (sex ratio. F:M 8:1) (Snooks *et al.*, 1985e). Most of these women have had children (Parks *et al.*, 1977; Snooks *et al.*, 1985b; Kiff and Swash 1984a) and many have experienced prolonged and difficult childbirth often necessitating forceps delivery.

Snooks *et al.* (1985e) assessed the anorectal function of 122 pregnant women and found the pudendal nerve terminal motor latency to be more markedly prolonged in multigravidae after vaginal delivery than in primigravidae. They also found that the fibre density in the external sphincter in the antenatal period was increased in multigravidae but not in primigravidae or nulliparous controls.

The risk of damage to the pudendal nerves is increased by the use of forceps during delivery (Snooks *et al.*, 1984) and high birth weight

(Snooks *et al.*, 1985e). Third degree perineal tears may render women incontinent due to direct injury to the pelvic floor muscles but may also be associated with pudendal nerve damage (Snooks *et al.*, 1985c).

An abnormal degree of perineal descent is present in many women 48–72 hours after vaginal delivery which is still present two months later (Snooks *et al.*, 1984). It is not present in women delivered by Caesarean section.

Pudendal nerve damage does not appear to be due to pregnancy but occurs during vaginal delivery. Snooks *et al.* (1984) suggested that the damage is reversible in 60% of cases. The internal sphincter appears to escape damage during childbirth (Snooks *et al.*, 1984).

Fourteen of the 24 multiparous women in the original study who had normal vaginal deliveries were re-examined in a follow up study. Snooks *et al.* (1990) found that five of these 14 women, five years after delivery, had clinical symptoms of stress incontinence.

The squeeze pressures of these multiparous women were lower in the antenatal period than in nulliparous women and after delivery fell further. Five years later the squeeze pressure had not recovered though perineal descent on defaecatory straining had resolved (Fig. 18).

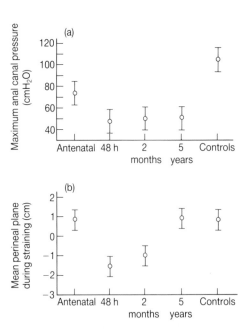

Fig. 18 (a) Maximal anal squeeze pressures (mean ± SEM) in multiparous women who were generally found to have lower pressures than age matched nulliparous controls and anal pressures did not return to the antenatal level when re-examined at the intervals shown after childbirth. (b) Mean position of the perineal plane during a maximum straining effort (mean ± SEM) in multiparous women around the time of delivery, (reproduced by permission of the publishers, Butterworth–Heinemann Ltd. from Snooks *et al.*, *Br J Surg*; 1990, **77**: 1359)

In the interval between the assessment at 48 hours after delivery and the reassessment at two months, PNTML improved but five years later the occult damage to the pudendal nerve had become more marked (Fig. 19). The fibre EMG had increased further at five years which suggests the continued presence of pudendal nerve dysfunction (Snooks *et al.*, 1990).

Cornes *et al.*, (1991), in another study, demonstrated a reduction in anal resting and squeeze pressures in the immediate post natal period. After six months resting pressure had returned to normal but squeeze pressure remained significantly reduced especially in patients who had a forceps delivery.

Anal sensation is impaired at all levels in the anal canal immediately after normal delivery or forceps delivery but only in the mid canal after delivery with the ventouse vacuum extractor. Cornes *et al.* (1991) have suggested that increased use of the ventouse instead of forceps could possibly reduce the risk of obstetric trauma to the sphincters and their innervation.

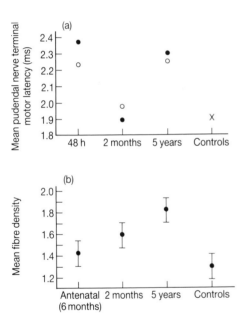

Fig. 19 (a) Pudendal nerve terminal motor latency in multiparous women around the time of childbirth demonstrating the increased latency in these women at their five year follow up. (Shaded circles for controls = the mean of right (unshaded boxes) and left (shaded boxes) data). (b) Single fibre electromyography of the external sphincter in multiparous women around the time of childbirth. Mean fibre density (± SEM) is increased at the five year follow up which is evidence of denervation and subsequent re-innervation of the muscle. (Reproduced by permission of the publishers, Butterworth–Heinemann Ltd. from Snooks *et al.*, *Br J Surg*; 1990, **77**: 1359)

Perineal descent (descending perineum syndrome)

Perineal descent is a common finding in patients with ano-rectal incontinence (Read *et al.*, 1984) and was present 69% of patients in one series (Snooks *et al.*, 1985b). Incontinence, however, is not related to the degree of descent in patients with the descending perineum syndrome (Bartolo *et al.*, 1983d).

The descending perineum syndrome is characterised by abnormal descent of the pelvic floor, which can be defined as descent of the anorectal angle to at least 2cm below the pubococcygeal line at rest, or at least 3cm on straining (Bartolo *et al.*, 1983d). The rectum is usually empty in these patients (Read *et al.*, 1986) but they experience the sensation of a lump in the anal canal and incomplete emptying at defaecation which may lead to frequent straining when the rectum is empty and possibly rectal ulceration (Rutter and Riddel, 1975).

Anal resting tone and maximum squeeze pressures are normal in continent patients with perineal descent but reduced in those who are incontinent (Read *et al.*, 1983; Bartolo *et al.*, 1983d). A lower volume of rectal distension is required to elicit the recto-anal inhibitory reflex in these patients (Bartolo *et al.*, 1983d; Read *et al.*, 1983) and the anorectal angle is increased (Bartolo *et al.*, 1983d; Read *et al.*, 1984; Womack *et al.*, 1986).

Histological examination has revealed hypertrophy of type 1 and type 2 fibres in the external sphincter in patients with the descending perineum syndrome which is consistent with damage to the nerve supply of the muscle (Henry *et al.*, 1982).

Patients with perineal descent and a long history of straining at stool have a prolonged pudendal nerve terminal motor latency (Kiff *et al.*, 1984). In patients with chronic constipation and defaecation straining, a delay in conduction from L1 to the external sphincter and to puborectalis has also been demonstrated (Snooks *et al.*, 1985a). Perineal descent during straining at stool appears therefore to damage the innervation of both of these muscles.

Lubowski *et al.* (1988c) measured PNTML before and after a maximal defaecation straining effort. They found that PNTML increases after straining in patients with perineal descent and that the difference between PNTML during and after straining was significantly correlated with the amount of perineal descent and with the position of the perineum after straining. The PNTML returned to the resting value within four minutes in all the subjects tested. These results support the concept that perineal descent causes pudendal nerve damage.

Incontinence in patients with the descending perineum syndrome is not necessarily secondary to the pudendal neuropathy. Anal resting tone is lower in incontinent patients with perineal descent than in continent patients with perineal descent. Internal anal sphincter weakness therefore appears to be an important factor leading to the development of incontinence in these patients (Bartolo *et al.*, 1983d; Womack *et al.*, 1986). This may also account for continence being maintained in some patients with perineal descent and evidence of pudendal neuropathy.

Rectal prolapse

Rectal prolapse is frequently accompanied by faecal incontinence. Anal resting pressure is reduced in these patients. Reduced squeeze pressures and increased fibre density in the external sphincter and puborectalis muscles have been found in patients with rectal prolapse and incontinence but not in patients with rectal prolapse alone (Neill *et al.*, 1981). Pudendal nerve terminal motor latency is also prolonged in patients with anorectal incontinence and rectal prolapse (Snooks *et al.*, 1985a).

Evidence of a neuropathy therefore is only present in the patients with rectal prolapse who are also incontinent of faeces. Rectal prolapse does not appear to be a cause of these neuropathic changes though there is clearly a deficiency in internal sphincter function as evidenced by the low resting pressures.

Effect of disease of the spinal cord or cauda equina

Nerve conduction to the external sphincter and pelvic floor muscles is abnormal in 73% of patients with anorectal incontinence (Snooks *et al.*, 1985d). In 23% of these patients there is a proximal conduction delay secondary to a cauda equina lesion. Both distal and proximal lesions may therefore be associated with faecal incontinence. The proximal lesions may account for the faecal incontinence that is seen in patients with neurological disease, e.g. spinal cord disease or multiple sclerosis. Sun and Read (1990) suggest that approximately 10% of their patients with anorectal incontinence have occult spinal lesions.

This subject will be discussed further later in this chapter.

Ageing and anorectal incontinence

It has been suggested that age related neurogenic factors may be important in the aetiology of faecal incontinence (Percy *et al.*, 1982; Read and Abouzekry, 1986). This subject will be considered in Chapter 7.

Anorectal sensory loss

Anal sensation

Anal sensation has been found to be impaired in a number of studies of faecally incontinent patients. Miller *et al.* (1987), using a water perfused thermode, found that the anal canal in normal subjects is highly sensitive to changes in temperature but this sensation is impaired in incontinent patients. Temperature sensation elsewhere in the body is known to play an important role in the distinction between gas, liquid and solid and is involved in the appreciation of 'wetness' (Vierck *et al.*, 1986).

Roe *et al.* (1986) demonstrated that anal mucosal electrosensitivity is also impaired in incontinent patients and this has been confirmed by Rogers *et al.* (1988) who found similar evidence in incontinent patients with pudendal motor neuropathy which suggests that there is a co-existent sensory neuropathy.

Miller *et al.* (1989) found significant impairment of anal sensation assessed by mucosal electrosensitivity and thermal sensitivity in incontinent patients compared with continent patients with proven perineal descent in the absence of changes in anal pressure or pudendal nerve terminal motor latency.

The sampling reflex is an important component of anal sensation which may be assessed by simultaneously measuring anal and rectal pressure. Miller *et al.* (1988) found that sampling occurs less frequently in incontinent patients (33%) than in controls (89%) and that the volume of rectal distension required to produce this is higher in the patients (median 40mls) than in the controls (median 10mls).

The results quoted above suggest that anal sensation is an important factor in faecal incontinence. Continence, however, is not always lost when anal sensation is abnormal or absent. Read and Read (1982) did not induce incontinence when they applied topical anaesthetic to the anus. Many paraplegic patients also maintain continence in the absence of anorectal sensation. Other continence mechanisms may compensate for the isolated loss of anal sensation but continence is lost when other deficiencies are also present, e.g. anal sphincter weakness.

Rectal sensation

The volume of rectal distension required to produce rectal sensation in normal subjects varies considerably. Most studies that have reported on rectal sensation from large groups of incontinent patients have not demonstrated any gross rectal sensory loss (Rogers *et al.*, 1988; Ferguson *et al.*, 1989).

There are, however, a small subgroup of incontinent patients in whom an abnormality of rectal sensation is the primary problem. Buser and Miner (1986) found that in 28% of the incontinent patients there was a delay in the sensation of rectal distension and that this tended to occur when the internal sphincter was already relaxed.

Lubowski and Nicholls (1988) identified eight (100%) patients without any evidence of anal sphincter muscle weakness or denervation in whom the threshold volume required to produce rectal sensation was significantly increxternal sphinctered. The mean volume required to produce the threshold of rectal sensation (143 mls) exceeded the threshold volume for the recto- anal reflex in the same patients (19 mls) by a considerable margin.

Sun *et al.*, (1990b) found that 10% of incontinent patients with normal anal pressures have abnormal rectal sensation. They exhibit a delay of at least two seconds between the onset of a sensory stimulus and its sensation. In this selected group of incontinent patients rectal sensory perception was followed by an increase in external anal sphincter activity.

A similar correlation was also observed between rectal sensation and rectal contractile activity. Internal sphincter relaxation occured in 11 (69%) of their patients before the onset of rectal sensation. During the study procedure, five (45%) of these patients leaked fluid from the anus. This leakage stopped once the subject perceived the sensation and contracted the external sphincter.

Internal sphincter weakness

The initial research on anorectal incontinence concentrated on the dysfunction and denervation of the external sphincter. Two thirds of patients with anorectal incontinence also have low anal resting pressures (Neill *et al.*, 1981) which suggests that there is internal sphincter dysfunction.

Internal sphincter weakness was initially dismissed as a contributory factor in anorectal incontinence (Corman, 1983; Swash, 1985) but its importance is now accepted.

In patients with the descending perineum syndrome (DPS) or rectal prolapse, the reduction in anal resting pressure is the main factor leading to faecal incontinence as anal squeeze pressure is reduced to the same degree in patients with DPS with faecal incontinence as in patients with DPS alone (Womack *et al.*, 1986) and similarly in patients with rectal prolapse (Frenckner and Ihre, 1976).

Prolonged anal sphincter recordings have generated useful information about the problem. Sun *et al.*, (1990c) demonstrated in a laboratory setting that incontinent patients exhibit more episodes of anal relaxation than control subjects, that anal pressure falls to a lower level and that fewer incontinent subjects exhibit a compensatory increase in external sphincter electrical activity. Sphincter relaxation occurs at lower volumes of balloon distension of the rectum in patients than in control subjects.

Sun *et al.* (1989) reported that 25% of patients with anorectal incontinence have internal sphincter weakness which fails to relax on rectal distension.

Kumar *et al.* (1989), using prolonged ambulatory recordings, have confirmed that spontaneous internal sphincter relaxation occurs more frequently and is of longer duration in patients with anorectal incontinence.

A strong correlation has been found between the anal endosonographic thickness of the internal sphincter and anal resting pressure. Law *et al.* (1990) used this technique to demonstrate that incontinent patients with low resting pressures have an abnormally thin internal sphincter.

Techniques have been developed to record internal sphincter smooth muscle EMG activity using either surface electrodes (Wankling *et al.*, (1968) or fine hooked wire electrodes (Duthie *et al.*, 1990).

Surface electrode recordings have shown that the internal sphincter slow wave activity (frequency 20–40/min) that is recordable in controls is often not recordable in incontinent patients (Lubowski *et al.*, 1988d) and that anal resting pressure and the frequency of internal sphincter smooth muscle activity is reduced in faecally incontinent patients (Duthie *et al.*, 1990).

Swash *et al.*, (1988) extensively investigated the internal anal sphincter in six patients with severe anorectal incontinence undergoing post anal repair and compared them with seven continent patients undergoing rectal excision for other causes. All of the patients and none of the controls had evidence of pudendal neuropathy. Electron microscopy was performed on biopsies taken from the lower edge of the internal sphincter during surgery. The internal sphincter was normal in six of the control subjects, with minor changes present in the other control subject. All of the patients showed varying degrees of atrophy and necrosis of smooth muscle cells which were separated by collagenised connective tissue.

There is still some uncertainty about the precise role of the internal sphincter in the pathophysiology of faecal incontinence. An abnormally weak internal sphincter could be expected to allow liquid faeces direct access to the anal canal which would deny the external sphincter sufficient time to respond to the entry of faeces into the rectum. It may also become desensitised to the continuous exposure to faeces. The reciprocal relationship between the contractile activities of the internal sphincter and the external sphincter is another important factor.

The external sphincter contracts to maintain continence when the internal sphincter is relaxed during rectal distension and similarly the internal sphincter preserves continence when the external sphincter is relaxed during micturition (Salducci *et al.*, 1982). Weakness of both muscles is therefore more likely to produce more severe incontinence than weakness of one muscle alone.

Read *et al.* (1984) demonstrated that patients incontinent to liquids had weakness of the internal sphincter. Patients who were incontinent of both solids and liquids had evidence of internal and external sphincter weakness. Patients incontinent to solids also had reduced or absent external sphincter contraction in response to rectal distension.

Rectal distension studies in incontinent patients have lead to the recognition of two distinct responses to rectal distension (Bannister *et al.*, 1989). Most incontinent patients exhibit a normal pattern of anal relaxation. Resting anal pressure profiles in these patients, however, differ from those in normal subjects as maximum anal canal pressure was found to be at the mid point of the anal canal instead of at the caudad pole which suggests a relative weakness of the external sphincter. This conclusion is also supportd by low anal squeeze pressure

The maximum reduction in anal pressure induced by rectal distension was similar in amplitude in this group of patients to that observed in the control group, implying normal internal sphincter tone, though the asymmetric profile of relaxation may suggest impaired tonic contraction of the sphincter in the outermost channels.

The remainder of Bannister *et al.*'s (1989) incontinent patients were older than the other incontinent patients and differed in a number of respects from the patients described above as they exhibit evidence of both external sphincter and internal sphincter dysfunction and tended to be incontinent of both liquids and solids. Anal relaxation did not occur in response to rectal distension. The low anal resting pressure in these patients excluded the possibility that they had Hirschsprungs disease (Aaronson and Nixon, 1972).

The abnormally weak internal sphincter makes little if any contribution to anal sphincter pressure. Rectal distension in these patients increases anal canal pressure in a pattern that resembles the profile of integrated electrical activity of the external anal sphincter. The external sphincter pressure and electrical activity response to rectal distension in this group of incontinent patients is similar in amplitude to the corresponding responses recorded in control subjects but the maximum squeeze pressure was found to be lower than in the other group of incontinent patients and normal controls. The maximum residual anal pressure during rectal distension, a measure of external sphincter tonic activity, was also reduced

Lubowski *et al.* (1988b) have assessed *in vitro* the response of the muscle strips obtained during surgery to noradrenaline and isoprenaline (to test myogenic tone) and the response to electrical field stimulation and dimethylphenylpiperazinium (to assess the activation of neural elements). All the muscle strips from the control subjects responded normally.

Strips of fresh internal sphincter muscle removed during post anal repair from patients with anorectal incontinence have shown pronounced pharmacological abnormalities (Speakman *et al.*, 1990; Lubowski *et al.*, 1988b).

Contractile sensitivity to noradrenaline is decreased in incontinent patients which suggests abnormal extrinsic alpha adrenergic innervation. The response to electrical field stimulation is also absent in many patients suggesting an abnormal intrinsic innervation. The latter is a non-adrenergic, non-cholinergic innervation whose activity is modified by the sympathetic extrinsic innervation. These pharmacological changes suggest that denervation may be important in causing internal sphincter dysfunction and provide a rationale for future drug management. Changes in resting pressure, electrical activity and spontaneous relaxations of the internal sphincter may also be due to an abnormality of the innervation of the sphincter.

Bannister *et al.*, (1989) discussed the possible causes of the observed internal sphincter weakness following their study, as none of their patients had diabetes mellitus or any other signs of autonomic dysfunction. Their patients, however, all had external sphincter weakness and abnormal descent of the pelvic floor. They suggested that the internal sphincter may require some structural support to maintain normal tone. If this is so, then possibly traction from the unsupported tissues of the pelvic floor could stretch the anus and cause apparent weakness. Another possible mechanism may involve stretch damage to the arteries or fragile autonomic nerves that supply the sphincter.

Lubowski *et al.*, (1988b), whilst accepting this suggestion, believe that internal anal sphincter dysfunction is more likely to be the result of autonomic dysfunction. Swash and Snooks' (1986) observations in patients with cauda equina lesions support this as internal anal sphincter function is normal even in the presence of advanced neuropathic damage to the external anal sphincter and pelvic floor musculature.

Diabetes

Faecal incontinence is a well recognised problem in patients with diabetes mellitus (Katz and Spiro, 1966). The gastrointestinal complications of diabetes are thought to be principally due to autonomic neuropathy (Scarpello and Sladen, 1978).

Schiller *et al.*, (1982) found that the onset of faecal incontinence in diabetic patients usually coincides with the onset of chronic diarrhoea. They found a significant reduction in internal sphincter pressure but not in external sphincter pressure in incontinent diabetics when compared with normal controls. Continent diabetic patients were found to have normal internal sphincter pressures even though 79% had symptoms suggestive of autonomic neuropathy. Schiller *et al.* suggest that the sphincter dysfunction in diabetic patients with faecal incontinence is due to a defect in either the autonomic innervation of the internal sphincter or in the smooth muscle itself. Diabetic autonomic neuropathy does not invariably cause internal sphincter dysfunction as evidenced by the presence of autonomic dysfunction in continent diabetics with normal anal resting pressure.

Rogers *et al.* (1988) compared the anorectal function of diabetic patients with peripheral neuropathy and normal bowel habit, patients with anorectal incontinence and a group of normal controls. They found that the anal pressures and pudendal nerve terminal motor latency in the diabetics was normal but they had neurophysiological evidence of neuropathy with increased anal canal mucosal electrosensitivity and increased external sphincter fibre density.

Wald and Tunuguntla (1984) found that the threshold volume at which diabetic patients with faecal incontinence experience rectal sensation was higher than in continent diabetics or non-diabetics with or without incontinence.

Minor degrees of pelvic floor neuropathy therefore do not appear to be associated with incontinence in diabetic patients. Incontinent diabetic patients, however, have been found to have impaired internal and external anal sphincter function and have a rectal sensory abnormality (Caruana *et al.*, 1991; Wald and Tunuguntla, 1984) (Figs 20 and 21).

Multiple sclerosis

Multiple sclerosis is another well recognised cause of both urinary and faecal incontinence. Population survey estimates of the prevalence of constipation or faecal incontinence among multiple sclerosis patients are between 39% and 68% (Caruana *et al.*, 1991). Hinds and Wald (1989), in a large population based study of multiple sclerosis patients, found that faecal incontinence had occurred at least once in the pre-ceding three months in 51% of their patients and in 13% it occurred weekly or more frequently.

Caruana *et al.* (1991) surprisingly found that the incontinent multiple sclerosis patients have a lower level of disability than continent multi-ple sclerosis patients and that the continent patients had a significantly higher threshold for the sensation of rectal sensation of distension than normal controls but not as marked as in the incontinent multiple sclerosis patients. Anal resting pressure was normal in both groups of multiple sclerosis patients but squeeze pressure was significantly reduced especially in the incontinent group (Figs. 20 and 21).

Disabled multiple sclerosis patients probably become constipated as a result of immobility, poor rectal sensation and abnormal colonic transit.

Spinal cord disease or injury

Urinary incontinence and constipation are common after traumatic spinal cord injury (Glick *et al.*, 1984).

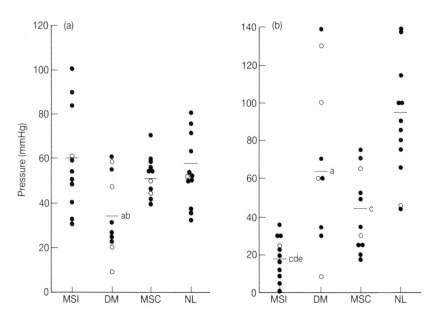

Fig. 20 Resting anal sphincter pressures (a) and maximal pressures (b) in the four groups of subjects. Mean resting pressures in the incontinent diabetics (DM) were significantly lower than in controls (NL), whereas they were normal in both MS groups. In contrast, maximal pressures were significantly lower in both MS groups and incontinent diabetics. Incontinent MS patients (MSI) had the most pronounced decrease, whereas continent MS patients (MSC) and incontinent diabetics had pressures intermediate between MSI and controls. ^aP <0.05 vs. NL; ^bP <0.02 vs. MSI; ^cP 0.01 vs. NL; ^dP <0.01 vs. MSC; ^eP <0.02 vs. DM; males; ● females. (Reproduced from Caruana et al., *Gastroenterology*; 1991, **100**: 468)

Early studies of patients with spinal cord injuries above the level of L1 revealed absent sensation of rectal distension (Frenckner, 1975; Wheatley *et al.*, 1977), poor anal resting pressure (Wheatley *et al.*, 1977), poor reflex contraction of the external sphincter in response to rectal distension (Frenckner 1975, Wheatley *et al.*, 1977) and impaired ability to retain a distended balloon within the rectum (Frenckner, 1975). Rectal compliance is decreased and ingestion of a meal does not necessarily produce a rectal response in these patients. The expected postprandial increase in colonic and rectal motility does not occur in patients with lesions above T12 who tend to suffer severe constipation (Aaronson *et al.*, 1985).

Sun *et al.* (1990a) assessed 20 incontinent patients with well defined incomplete spinal lesions and found that patients with high spinal lesions i.e. above T12, had normal anal resting pressure but abnormally low squeeze pressure and impaired rectal sensation. They also demonstrated that exaggerated external anal sphincter responses to rectal distension and to increases in intra-abdominal pressure occur in these patients.

In normal individuals rectal sensation and external sphincter activity are closely linked to each other and both occur when rectal contractions are stimulated by distension. In high spinal lesion patients this relationship is absent and may therefore fail to occur when continence is threatened.

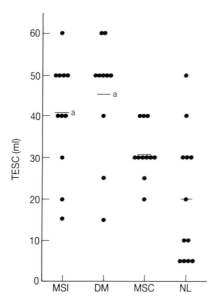

Fig. 21 Thresholds of phasic external anal sphincter contraction (TESC) in response to rectal distention in the four groups of subjects. Both incontinent MS patients (MSI) and diabetics (DM) had significantly higher thresholds than did control subjects (NL), whereas continent MS patients (MSC) had no significant differences from controls. [a]*P* <0.05 vs. NL. (Reproduced from Caruana *et al.*, *Gastroenterology*; 1991, **100**: 468)

Patients with low spinal lesions, i.e. L1 or below, have low resting pressures, low squeeze pressures and poor rectal sensation. Their external sphincter responses to rectal distension and increased intra-abdominal pressure are also impaired.

Patients with a mixture of high and low spinal lesions have the lowest resting and squeeze pressures and have no conscious or reflex external sphincter activity. They leak during rectal distension and during increases in intra-abdominal pressure.

In the absence of overt spinal cord disease 23% of young women with anorectal incontinence who had spinal stimulation studies performed by Snooks *et al.* (1985d) were found to have evidence of delayed proximal nerve conduction to the external sphincter, which suggests occult abnormalities in the spinal cord or nerve roots.

References

Aaronson MJ, Freed MM, Burakof R. (1985) Colonic myoelectric activity in persons with spinal cord injury. *Dig Dis Sci*; **30**: 295–300.

Aaronson J, Nixon HH. (1972) A clinical reevaluation of anorectal pressure studies in the diagnosis of Hirschsprung's Disease. *Gut*; **13**: 138–46.

Bannister JJ, Read NW, Donnelly TC, Sun WM. (1989) External and internal anal sphincter responses to rectal distension in normal subjects and in patients with idiopathic faecal incontinence. *Br J Surg*; **76**: 617–21.

Bartolo DCC, Jarratt JA, Read NW. (1983a) The cutaneo-anal reflex: a useful index of neuropathy? *Br J Surg*; **70**: 660–3.

Bartolo DCC, Jarratt JA, Read NW. (1983b) The use of conventional electromyography to assess external sphincter neuropathy in man. *J Neurol Neurosurg Psychiat*; **46**: 1115–18.

Bartolo DCC, Jarratt JA, Read MG, Donnelly TC, Read NW. (1983c) The role of partial denervation of the puborectalis muscle in idiopathic faecal incontinence. *Br J Surg*; **70**: 664–7.

Bartolo DCC, Read NW, Jarratt JA, Read MG, Donnelly TC, Johnson AG. (1983d) Differences in anal sphincter function and clinical presentation in patients with pelvic floor descent. *Gastroenterology*; **85**: 68–75.

Beersiek F, Parks AG, Swash M. (1979) Pathogenesis of ano-rectal incontinence. A histometric study of the anal sphincter musculature. *J Neurol Sci*; **42**: 111–27.

Buser WD, Miner PB. (1986) Delayed rectal sensation with faecal incontinence. Successful treatment using anorectal manometry. *Gastroenterology*; **91**: 1186–91.

Caruana BJ, Wald A, Hinds JP, Eidelman BH. (1991) Anorectal sensory and motor function in neurogenic fecal incontinence. Comparison between multiple sclerosis and diabetes mellitus. *Gastroenterology*; **100**: 465–70.

Corman ML. (1983) The management of anal incontinence. *Surg Clin N America*; **63**: 177–92.

Cornes H, Bartolo DCC, Stirrat GM. (1991) Changes in anal canal sensation after childbirth. *Br J Surg*; **78**: 74–7.

Duthie GS, Miller R, Bartolo DCC. (1990) Internal anal sphincter electromyographic frequency is related to anal canal resting pressure. Both are reduced in idiopathic faecal incontinence. *Gut*; **31**: A619.

Felt Bersma RJF, Klinkenberg-Knol EC, Meuwissen SGM. (1990) Anorectal function investigations in incontinent and continent patients. *Dis Colon Rectum*; **33**: 479–86.

Ferguson GH, Redford J, Barrett JA, Kiff ES. (1989) The appreciation of rectal distension in faecal incontinence. *Dis Colon Rectum*; **32**: 964–7.

Frenckner B. (1975) Function of the anal sphincters in spinal man. *Gut*; **16**: 638–44.

Frenckner B, Ihre T. (1976) Function of the anal sphincters in patients with intussusception of the rectum. *Gut*; **17**: 147–51.

Glick ME, Meshkinpour H, Haldiman S, Hoehler F, Downey N, Bradley WE. (1984) Colonic dysfunction in patients with thoracic spinal cord injury. *Gastroenterology*; **86**: 287–94.

Hardcastle JD, Parks AG. (1970) A study of anal incontinence and some principles of surgical treatment. *Proc Roy Soc Med*; **63**: 116–18.

Henry MM, Parks AG, Swash M. (1980) The anal reflex in idiopathic faecal incontinence; an electrophysiological study. *Br J Surg*; **67**: 781–3.

Henry MM, Parks AG, Swash M. (1982) The pelvic floor musculature in the descending perineum syndrome. *Br J Surg*; **69**: 470–2.

Henry MM, Swash M. (1978) Assessment of pelvic floor disorders and incontinence by electrophysiological recording of the anal reflex. *Lancet*; i: 1290–1.

Hinds JP, Wald A. (1989) Colonic and anorectal dysfunction associated with multiple sclerosis. *Am J Gastroenterology*; **84**: 587–95.

Katz LA, Spiro HM. (1966) Gastrointestinal manifestations of diabetes. *New Eng J Med*; **275**: 594–624.

Kiff ES, Barnes PRH, Swash M. (1984) Evidence of pudendal neuropathy in patients with perineal descent and chronic straining at stool. *Gut*; **25**: 1279–82.

Kiff ES, Swash M. (1984a) Slowed conduction in the pudendal nerves in idiopathic (neurogenic) faecal incontinence. *Br J Surg*; **71**: 614–16.

Kiff ES, Swash M. (1984b) Normal proximal and delayed distal conduction in the pudendal nerves of patients with idiopathic (neurogenic) faecal incontinence. *J Neurol Neurosurg Psychiat*; **47**: 820–3.

Kumar D, Williams NS, Waldron D, Wingate DL. (1989) Prolonged manometric recording of anorectal motor activity in ambulant human subjects: evidence of periodic activity. *Gut*; **30**: 1007–11.

Law PJ, Kamm MA, Bartram CI. (1990) A comparison between electromyography and anal endosonography in mapping external anal sphincter defects. *Dis Colon Rectum*; **33**: 370–3.

Law PJ, Kamm MA, Bartram CI. (1991) Anal endosonography in the investigation of faecal incontinence. *Br J Surg*; **78**: 312–14.

Lubowski DZ, Jones PN, Swash M, Henry MM. (1988a) Asymmetrical pudendal nerve damage in pelvic floor disorders. *Int J Colorect Dis*; **3**: 158–60.

Lubowski DZ, Nicholls RJ. (1988c) Faecal incontinence associated with reduced pelvic sensation. *Br J Surg*; **75**: 1086–8.

Lubowski DZ, Nicholls RJ, Burleigh DE, Swash M. (1988b) Internal anal sphincter in neurogenic faecal incontinence. *Gastroenterology*; **95**: 997–1002.

Lubowski DZ, Swash M, Nicholls RJ, Henry MM. (1988c) Increase in pudendal nerve terminal motor latency with defaecation straining. *Br J Surg*; **75**: 1095–7.

Marsden CD, Merton PA, Morton HB. (1982) The latency of the anal reflex. *J Neurol Neurosurg Psychiat*; **45**: 857.

Matheson DM, Keighley MRB. (1981) Manometric evaluation of rectal prolapse and faecal incontinence. *Gut*; **22**: 126–9.

Miller R, Bartolo DCC, Cervero F, Mortensen NJMcC. (1987) Anorectal temperature sensation: a comparison of normal and incontinent patients. *Br J Surg*; **74**: 511–15.

Miller R, Bartolo DCC, Cervero F, Mortensen NJMcC. (1988) Anorectal sampling: a comparison of normal and incontinent patients. *Br J Surg*; **75**: 44–7.

Miller R, Bartolo DCC, Cervero F, Mortensen NJMcC. (1989) Differences in anal sensation in continent and incontinent patients with perineal descent. *Int J Colorect Dis*; **4**: 45–9.

Neill ME, Parks AG, Swash M. (1981) Physiological studies of the anal sphincter musculature in faecal incontinence and rectal prolapse. *Br J Surg*; **68**: 531–6.

Neill ME, Swash M. (1980) Increased motor unit fibre density in the external anal sphincter in ano-rectal incontinence: a single fibre EMG study. *J Neurol Neurosurg Psychiat*; **43**: 343–7.

Parks AG. (1967) Post-anal perineorrhaphy for rectal prolapse. *Proc Roy Soc Med*; **60**: 920–1.

Parks AG. (1975) Anorectal incontinence. *Proc Roy Soc Med*; **68**: 681–90.

Parks AG, Swash M, Urich H. (1977) Sphincter denervation in anorectal incontinence and rectal prolapse. *Gut*; **18**: 656–65.

Pedersen E, Harving H, Klemar B, Torring J. (1978) Human anal reflexes. *J Neurol Neurosurg Psychia*; **41**: 813–18.

Pedersen E, Klemar B, Schroder HD, Torring J. (1982) Anal sphincter responses after perianal electrical stimulation. *J Neurol Neurosurg Psychiat*; **45**: 770–3.

Percy JP, Neill ME, Kandiah TK, Swash M. (1982) A neurogenic factor in faecal incontinence in the elderly. *Age and Ageing*; **11**: 175–9.

Porter NH. (1962) A physiological study of the pelvic floor in rectal prolapse. *Ann Roy Coll Surg Eng*; **31**: 379–404.

Read MG, Read NW. (1982) Role of anorectal sensation in preserving continence. *Gut*; **23**: 345–7.

Read NW, Abouzekry L. (1986) Why do patients with faecal impaction have faecal incontinence? *Gut*; **27**: 283–7.

Read NW, Bartolo DCC, Read MG. (1984) Differences in anal function in patients with incontinence to solids and in patients with incontinence to liquids. *Br J Surg*; **71**: 39–42.

Read NW, Bartolo DCC, Read MG, Hall J, Haynes WG, Johnson AG. (1983) Differences in anorectal manometry between patients with haemorrhoids and patients with descending perineum syndrome: implications for management. *Br J Surg*; **70**: 656–9.

Read NW, Harford WV, Schmulen AC, Read MG, Santa Ana CA, Fordtran JS. (1979) A clinical study of patients with faecal incontinence and diarrhoea. *Gastroenterology*; **76**: 747–56.

Read NW, Timms JM, Barfield LJ, Donnelly TC, Bannister JJ. (1986) Impairment of defaecation in young women with severe constipation. *Gastroenterology*. **90**: 53–60.

Roe AM, Bartolo DCC, Mortensen NJMcC. (1986) New method for assessment of anal sensation in various anorectal disorders. *Br J Surg*; **73**: 310–12.

Rogers J, Levy DM, Henry MM, Misiewicz JJ. (1988) Pelvic floor neuropathy: a comparative study of diabetes mellitus and idiopathic faecal incontinence. *Gut*; **29**: 756–61.

Rossolimo G. (1891) Der anal reflex, seine physiologie und pathologie. *Neurologisches Centralblatt*; **10**: 257–9.

Rutter KRP, Riddell RH. (1975) The solitary ulcer syndrome of the rectum. *Clin Gastroenterology*; **4**: 505–30.

Salducci J, Planche D, Naudy B. (1982) Physiological role of the internal anal sphincter and the external anal sphincter during micturition. in Weinbeck M, (ed) *Motility of the Digestive Tract*. Raven Press, New York.

Scarpello JHB, Sladen GE. (1978) Diabetes and the gut. *Gut*; **19**: 1153–62.

Schiller LR, Santa Ana CA, Schmulen AC, Hendler RS, Harford WV, Fordtran JS. (1982) Pathogenesis of fecal incontinence in diabetes mellitus. Evidence for internal anal sphincter dysfunction. *New En J Med*; **307**: 1666–71.

Schwartz MS, Sargeant MK, Swash M. (1976) Longitudinal fibre splitting in neurogenic muscular disorders; its relation to the pathogenesis of 'myopathic' change. *Brain*; **99**: 617–36.

Snooks SJ, Barnes PRH, Swash M, Henry MM. (1985a) Damage to the innervation of the pelvic floor musculature in chronic constipation. *Gastroenterology*; **89**: 977–81.

Snooks SJ, Henry MM, Swash M. (1985b) Anorectal incontinence and rectal prolapse: differential assessment of the innervation to puborectalis and external anal sphincter muscles. *Gut*; **26**: 470–6.

Snooks SJ, Henry MM, Swash M. (1985c) Faecal incontinence due to external anal sphincter division in childbirth is associated with damage to the innervation of the pelvic floor musculature: a double pathology. *Br J Obstet Gynaecol*; **92**: 824–8.

Snooks SJ, Setchell M, Swash M, Henry MM. (1984) Injury to the innervation of the pelvic floor musculature in childbirth. *Lancet*; **ii**: 546–50.

Snooks SJ, Swash M, Henry MM. (1985d) Abnormalities in central and peripheral nerve conduction in patients with anorectal incontinence. *J Roy Soc Med*; **78**: 294–300.

Snooks SJ, Swash M, Henry MM, Setchell M. (1985e) Risk factors in childbirth causing damage to the pelvic floor innervation. *Br J Surg*; **72** (Suppl): S15–S17.

Snooks SJ, Swash M, Mathers SE, Henry MM. (1990) Effect of vaginal delivery on the pelvic floor: a 5-year follow up. *Br J Surg*; **77**: 1358–60.

Speakman CTM, Hoyle CHV, Kamm MA, Henry MM, Nicholls RJ, Burnstock G. (1990) Adrenergic control of the internal anal sphincter is abnormal in patients with idiopathic faecal incontinence. *Br J Surg*; **77**: 134–44.

Speakman CTM, Burnett SJD, Kamm MA, Bartram CI. (1991) Sphincter injury after anal dilatation demonstrated by anal endosonography. *Br J Surg*; **78**: 1429–30.

Stalberg E, Thiele B. (1975) Motor unit fibre density in the extensor digitorum communis muscle. *J Neurol Neurosurg Psychiat*; **38**: 874–80.

Stalberg E, Trontelj JV. (1979) *Single Fibre electromyography*. The Mirvalle Press Ltd, Old Woking, Surrey.

Sun WM, Read NW. (1990) Occult spinal lesions: a common undetected cause of faecal incontinence. *Lancet*; **335**: 166.

Sun WM, Read NW, Donnelly TC. (1989) Impaired internal anal sphincter in a subgroup of patients with idiopathic faecal incontinence. *Gastroenterology*; **97**: 130–5.

Sun WM, Read NW, Donnelly TC. (1990a) Anorectal function in incontinent patients with cerebrospinal disease. *Gastroenterology*; **99**: 1372–9.

Sun WM, Read NW, Miner PB. (1990b) Relation between rectal sensation and anal function in normal subjects and patients with faecal incontinence. *Gut*; **31**: 1056–61.

Sun WM, Read NW, Miner PB, Kerrigan DD, Donnelly TC. (1990c) The role of transient internal sphincter relaxation in faecal incontinence? *Int J Colorect Dis*; **5**: 31–6.

Swash M. (1980) Idiopathic faecal incontinence: Histopathological evidence on pathogenesis. In Wright R (ed) *Recent Advances in Gastrointestinal Pathology*. pp. 71–89. W.B. Saunders, Philadelphia.

Swash M. (1982) Early and late components of the human anal reflex. *J Neurol Neurosurg Psychiat*; **45**: 767–9.

Swash M. (1985) New concepts in incontinence. *Br Med J*; **290**: 4–5.

Swash M, Snooks SJ. (1986) Slowed motor conduction in lumbosacral nerve roots in cauda equina lesions: a new diagnostic technique. *J Neurol Neurosurg Psychiat*; **49**: 808–16.

Swash M, Gray A, Lubowski DZ, Nicholls RJ. (1988) Ultrastructural changes in internal anal sphincter in neurogenic faecal incontinence. *Gut*; **29**: 1692–1698.

Vierck CJ, Greenspan JD, Ritz LA, Yeomans DC. (1986) The spinal pathways contributing to the ascending conduction and descending modulation of pain sensation and reactions. In: Yaksh TL (ed) *Spinal Afferent Processing*, pp. 275–329. Plenum Press, New York.

Vodusek DB, Janko M, Lokar J. (1983) Direct and reflex responses in perineal muscles on electrical stimulation. *J Neurol Neurosurg Psychiat*; **46**: 67–71.

Wald A, Tunuguntla AK. (1984) Anorectal sensorimotor dysfunction in faecal incontinence and diabetes mellitus. Modification with biofeedback therapy. *New Eng J Med*; **310**: 1282–7.

Wankling WJ, Brown BH, Collins CD, Duthie HL. (1968) Basic electrical activity in the anal canal in man. *Gut*; **9**: 459–60.

Wheatley IC, Hardy KJ, Dent J. (1977) Anal pressure studies in spinal patients. *Gut*; **18**: 488–90.

Womack NR, Morrison JFB, Williams NS. (1986) The role of pelvic floor denervation in the aetiology of idiopathic faecal incontinence. *Br J Surg*; **73**: 404–7.

Wright AL, Williams NS, Gibson JS, Neal DE, Morrison JFB. (1985) Electrically evoked activity in the human external anal sphincter. *Br J Surg*; **72**: 38–41.

7

Ageing and anorectal function

A number of age related changes in anorectal function have recently been identified which may account for the high prevalence of anorectal problems in the elderly.

Ageing and bowel habit

The frequency of bowel movements in normal individuals has been found to be between three times per day and three times per week (Connell *et al.*, 1965; Rendtorff and Kashigarian, 1966; Milne and Williamson, 1972). Ageing does not appear to lead to any change in the frequency of defaecation (Connell *et al.*, 1965).

An age associated increase in the use of laxatives, especially among aged females, has been described (Connell *et al.* 1965; Milne and Williamson, 1972). Connell *et al.*, (1965) interviewed patients in general practitioners waiting rooms and found that 30% of the over 60s were regular laxative users (once weekly or more) compared with 6% of the under-40s and 18% of those aged betwen 40 and 59 years. Milne and Williamson (1972), in a community survey, found that more than 50% of males and females aged over 70 years use a laxative at least once per week. Over 60% of their study subjects passed at least one stool per day.

Moore-Gillon (1984), in a study of 350 people attending an ear, nose and throat outpatient department, found that laxatives had been used in the previous year by 32% of females and 16% of males. Twenty five percent of both sexes thought that regular purgation was beneficial, even if bowel function was quite regular, and 9% of females and 20% of males thought it was harmful if the bowels were not opened every day.

Laxatives appear to be taken regularly by many elderly people who are not constipated. They were children during a period at the beginning of this century when the medical profession considered auto-intoxication from the colon to be the cause of a large number of medical ailments (Lane, 1915). Many eminent surgeons performed colectomies to overcome its ill-effects. It is not surprising therefore that the practice of purgation at least once per week was widely undertaken.

Colonic motility and ageing

Colorectal motility in old age has not been the subject of much study and no studies have been performed utilising the modern assessment techniques that are now available.

In healthy elderly people, whole gut transit time has been found to be normal (Eastwood, 1972) as has colonic motility (Loening-Baucke and Anuras, 1984a). Atrophy of colonic muscle was described in an early study (Yamagata, 1965) but this does not fit with the observations of transit time.

The effect of age on anal resting pressure

It is generally agreed that there is a wide range of anal resting pressure in normal individuals. Studies that have reported upon the effect of age on anal resting pressure have not produced consistent results. A reduction in resting pressure with increasing age has been reported from a number of studies (Read *et al.*, 1979, 1985; Bannister *et al.*, 1987; McHugh and Diamant 1987). Matheson and Keighley (1981), however, only demonstrated low resting pressures in very old people and Loening-Baucke and Anuras (1984b) did not find any age related pressure change.

The most recent studies have not found any correlation between resting pressure and age in normal individuals (Barrett *et al.*, 1989; Laurberg and Swash 1989).

The effect of age on the external anal sphincter and its innervation

There is no dispute that external anal sphincter pressure, i.e. squeeze pressure, decreases with age ((Read *et al.*, 1979; Bannister *et al.*, 1987; Matheson and Keighley, 1981; McHugh and Diamant, 1987; Barrett *et al.*, 1989; Laurberg and Swash, 1989). Two of these studies have also investigated data on the innervation of the external sphincter in old age (Barrett *et al.*, 1989; Laurberg and Swash, 1989).

Laurberg and Swash studied 121 subjects (84% female) aged between 20 and 80 years who were awaiting sphincter saving surgery for inflammatory bowel disease or anorectal carcinoma. They found that the decline in anal squeeze pressure mostly occurs in the fifth and sixth decades (Fig. 22). Pressures were higher in men than in women at all ages. There is greater variability in squeeze pressures in older women than in older men. The resting position of the perineal plane was also found to be lower in older women but no age related change was detected in men. Squeeze pressure in elderly women does not, however, appear to be related to parity (McHugh and Diamant, 1987).

Barrett *et al.* (1989) studied 88 subjects with normal bowel habit; 57 young healthy volunteers (mean age 48 years) were compared with 31 elderly outpatients attending a geriatric day hospital (mean age 77 years). They found the squeeze pressures to be considerably lower in the elderly patients (mean 51 cmH_2O) than in the younger subjects (mean 167 cmH_2O) (Fig. 23).

A number of age related changes in striated muscle are well recognised. Muscle strength (Burke *et al.*, 1953; Campbell *et al.*, 1973; Grimby and Saltin, 1983; Pearson *et al*, 1985; Larsson, 1978, 1982; Danneskiold-Samson *et al.*, 1984; Davies *et al.*, 1986) and muscle mass (Young *et al.*, 1985; Imamura *et al.*, 1983; Lexell *et al.*, 1983; Grimby and Saltin, 1983; Danneskiold-Samson *et al.*, 1984) both decline in old age. Elderly muscle contracts more slowly and is more easily fatigued than that of younger subjects (Davies *et al.*, 1986) and there is a reduction in muscle blood flow during muscle contraction (Barcroft and Millen, 1939; Edwards *et al.*, 1972).

These effects may be primarily due to changes within muscles themselves but muscle will also reflect changes in other parts of the motor unit (neuromuscular junction, peripheral nerve or anterior horn cell)

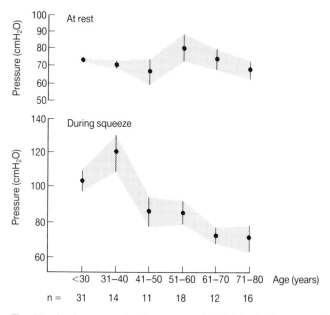

Fig. 22 Anal manometry from normal individuals demonstrating the absence of a relationship between age and resting pressure but a fall in squeeze pressure after the fourth decade. (Reproduced from Laurberg and Swash, *Dis Colon Rectum*; 1989, **32**: 739)

and those structures may in turn be influenced by degeneration in higher centres of the nervous system.

Histological evidence of denervation has been described in a number of studies of ageing muscle (Tomlinson *et al.*, 1969; Tomonaga, 1977; Grimby and Saltin, 1983).

Electrophysiological studies have shown a progressive fall in the number of functioning motor units after the age of 60 years in several different muscles (Campbell *et al.*, 1973, Sica *et al.*, 1974) and there is also evidence to suggest that the remaining motor units enlarge to re-innervate the muscle fibres that have lost their own nerve supply (Campbell *et al.*, 1973; Stalberg and Thiele, 1975; Stalberg and Trontelj, 1979; Rosenfalck, 1975; Grimby and Saltin, 1983) which is consistent with denervation muscle atrophy.

There is also evidence in ageing muscle of type 2 fibre atrophy

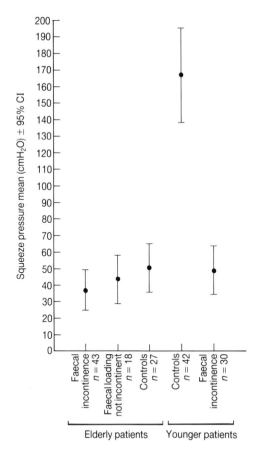

Fig. 23 Comparison of anal squeeze pressures (mean ± 95% confidence interval) between elderly and younger faecally incontinent patients and their controls. (Data from Barrett *et al.*, 1989)

(Larsson, 1983) and a decrease in the synthesis and release of neurotransmitter and neurotrophic agents with increasing age (Gutman, 1974).

Electrophysiological studies have produced clear evidence of denervation and re-innervation of the external anal sphincter in old age. Concentric needle EMG studies revealed an increase in the mean duration of motor unit potentials (Bartolo *et al.*, 1983) and increased fibre density has been demonstrated in studies using single fibre EMG (Neill and Swash, 1980; Percy *et al.*, 1982; Laurberg and Swash, 1989).

The ageing process has been considered as a possible cause of this denervation. Morphological studies of ageing human peripheral nerve have revealed a reduction in the density of myelinated and unmyelinated nerve fibres with increasing age (Lascelles and Thomas, 1966; Ochoa and Mair, 1969; Arnold and Harriman, 1970; Jacobs and Love, 1985).

Motor and sensory nerve conduction velocity slows after approximately 60 years (Wagman and Lesse, 1952; Buchthal and Rosenfalck, 1966) particularly in the distal parts of axons (Dorfman and Bosley, 1979; Taylor, 1984). Swash and Schwartz (1981) considered that distal motor latency is increased in most nerves in the elderly, especially in the hand. Rosenfalck (1975), however, did not find nerve conduction velocity to be reduced in all nerves in old age.

Pudendal neuropathy is now well recognised as a cause of external sphincter weakness in younger patients with anorectal incontinence. Pudendal neuropathy can be detected by measuring pudendal nerve terminal motor latency (PNTML).

Barrett *et al.* (1989), using this technique did not detect any age related difference in mean PNTML between their groups of young (2.0 ms. 95% CI 1.9–2.2) and elderly control subjects (2.1 ms. 95% CI 1.9–2.2). No correlation was found between age and PNTML.

Laurberg and Swash (1989) also measured PNTML in their study patients. They concluded that PNTML was affected by age. Their results do not, however, appear to support this conclusion. They found the mean PNTML in women aged over 50 years to be 2.15 ms (sd 0.3). The mean PNTML in younger women was 2.0 ms (sd 0.2). They suggest that this difference is significant but this data does not appear significantly different. They comment that there is a greater degree of variability in older women but no linear relationship was detected between PNTML and age.

It appears, therefore, that ageing does not affect pudendal nerve terminal motor latency and therefore the observed weakness of the external sphincter in the elderly is not due to damage of the distal part of the pudendal nerve. Age related loss of anterior horn cells or motor nerve fibres from the proximal innervation of the external sphincter cannot be excluded by these results. There is evidence to suggest that this may occur with increasing age, as Duncan (1934) found a reduced number of ventral root fibres in rats aged 800 days, and Gardner (1940) found a 27% reduction in the number of nerve fibres in the ventral roots at the T8 and T9 levels in subjects aged 70 to 79 years.

Laurberg and Swash (1989) discussed other possible causes of low anal squeeze pressures. They suggested that the menopause may be a significant factor especially as the difference observed in females was not present in the males studied. There is some evidence of a hormone dependent factor in the pelvic floor musculature. Histometric studies have demonstrated that the type 1 muscle fibres in levator ani are larger than the type 2 fibres (Beersiek *et al.*, 1979). This is the reverse of the normal relationship of these histochemical fibre types in all other striated muscles studied in men or women (Polgar *et al.*, 1973).

The loss of anterior horn cells which occurs in old age is not likely to be the cause of the low external sphincter pressures observed in middle age.

Barrett *et al.* (1989) also found an association between anal squeeze pressure and mobility. The least mobile patients in the study had the lowest squeeze pressures (Fig. 24) which suggests that atrophy of skeletal muscle and the external sphincter may occur together due to a common underlying neurological abnormality.

Ageing and the recto-anal reflex

The reflex activity of the external anal sphincter is also impaired in old age. The normal recto-anal reflex was described on p. 35. Barrett *et al.* (1989) reported that reflex contraction of the external anal sphincter in response to rectal distension (inflation reflex) was absent in 59% of their elderly control patients, though Read and Abouzekry (1986) had demonstrated it in 80% of their elderly control group. A higher incidence of neurological disease in the former study may account for this difference. The reflex is known to be absent in paraplegic patients with lesions above the level of L1 (Frenckner, 1975; Wheatley *et al.*, 1977).

Bannister *et al.*, (1987) studied the recto-anal inhibitory reflex and suggested that lower volumes of rectal distension are required to inhibit anal sphincter tone in the elderly. Barrett *et al.* (1989) were able to elicit the inhibitory reflex in 82% of their elderly control patients.

The effect of age on rectal sensation

Data is available on rectal sensation in old age from two studies. Bannister *et al.* (1987) found that the rectal volume required to produce the sensation of a 'call to stool' was greater in their elderly subjects than in their younger subjects. The rectal pressures at each level of sensation were, however, similar in both age groups which suggests that rectal sensation is mediated by tension or pressure receptors.

Barrett *et al.* (1990), however, found the mean rectal volume to produce the call to stool was 88mls (range 30–250) in the elderly compared with 78mls (range 40–150) in their younger subjects. There was no difference in the rectal pressures measured when the call

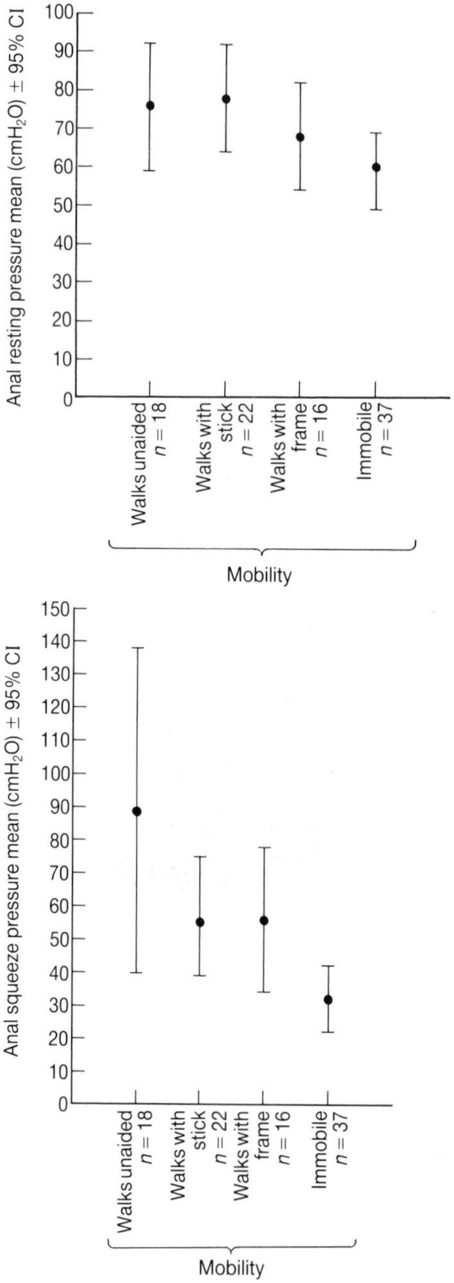

Fig. 24 Comparison of anal resting and squeeze pressures (mean ± 95% confidence interval) in elderly patients on the basis of their level of mobility. A relationship is demonstrated between mobility and squeeze pressure. (Data from Barrett *et al.,* 1989)

to stool was experienced. It would appear unlikely, therefore, that there is any significant change in this rectal sensation with normal ageing.

Ageing and defaecation

Defaecation does not appear to be affected by normal ageing as nearly all the normal elderly subjects studied by Bannister *et al.* (1987) were able to defaecate simulated stools within five minutes. They also found that the anorectal angle does not differ between young and elderly subjects.

Ageing and anal sensation

The age related changes that occur in anal sensation will be discussed in Chapter 9.

References

Arbuthnot Lane (1915) see Lane WA. (1915)

Arnold N, Harriman DGF. (1970) The incidence of abnormality in control human peripheral nerves studied by single axon dissection. *J Neurol Neurosurg Psychiat*; **33**: 55–61.

Bannister JJ, Abouzekry L, Read NW. (1987) Effect of aging on anorectal function. *Gut*; **28**: 353–7.

Barcroft H, Millen JLE. (1939) The blood flow through muscle during sustained contraction. *J Physiol (London)*; **97**: 17–31.

Barrett JA, Brocklehurst JC, Kiff ES, Ferguson G, Faragher EB. (1989) Anal function in geriatric patients with faecal incontinence. *Gut*; **30**: 1244–51.

Barrett JA, Brocklehurst JC, Kiff ES, Ferguson G, Faragher EB. (1990) Rectal motility studies in geriatric patients with faecal incontinence. *Age and Ageing*. **19**: 311–17.

Bartolo DCC, Jarratt JA, Read NW. (1983) The use of conventional electromyography to assess external sphincter neuropathy in man. *J Neurol Neurosurg Psychiat*; **46**: 1115–18.

Beersiek F, Parks AG, Swash M. (1979) Pathogenesis of ano-rectal incontinence. A histometric study of the anal sphincter musculature. *J Neurol Sci*; **42**: 111–27.

Buchthal F, Rosenfalck P. (1966) Evoked action potentials and conduction velocity in human sensory nerves. *Brain Res*; **3**: 1–122.

Burke WE, Tuttle WW, Thompson CW, Janney CD, Webber RJ. (1953) The relation of grip strength and grip strength endurance to age. *J Appl Physiol*; **5**: 628–30.

Campbell MJ, McComas AJ, Petito F. (1973) Physiological basis of ageing in muscles. *J Neurol Neurosurg Psychiat*; **36**: 174–82.

Connell AM, Hilton C, Irvine G, Lennard-Jones JE, Misiewicz JJ. (1965) Variation of bowel habit in two population samples. *Br Med J*; **2**: 1095–9.

Danneskiold-Samson B, Kofod V, Munter J, Grimby G, Schohr P, Jensen G. (1984) Muscle strength and functional capacity in 78–81 year old men and women. *Eur J Appl Physiol*; **52**: 310–14.

Davies CTM, Thomas DO, White MJ. (1986) Mechanical properties of young and elderly human muscle. *Acta Med Scand.* (Suppl); **711**: 219–26.

Dorfman LJ, Bosley TM. (1979) Age related changes in peripheral and central nerve conduction in man. *Neurology*; **29**: 38–44.

Duncan D. (1934) A determination of the number of nerve fibres in the 8th thoracic and largest lumbar ventral roots of the albino rat. *J Compar Neurol*; **59**: 47–60.

Eastwood HDH. (1972) Bowel transit studies in the elderly: radioopaque markers in the investigation of constipation. *Gerontol Clin*; **14**: 154–9

Edwards RHT, Hill DK, McDonnell M. (1972) Myothermal and intramuscular pressure measurements during anaerobic contractions of the human quadriceps muscle. *J Physiol* (London); **224**: 58P–59P.

Frenckner B. (1975) Function of the anal sphincters in spinal man. *Gut*; **16**: 638–44.

Gardner E. (1940) Decrease in human neurones with age. *Anat Record*; **77**: 529–36.

Grimby G, Saltin B. (1983) Mini-review. The ageing muscle. *Clin Physiol*; **3**: 209–18.

Gutman E. (1974) Age changes in the neuromuscular system and aspects of rehabilitation medicine. In Buerger AA *et al.* (eds) *Neurophysiologic Aspects of Rehabilitation Medicine*. Charles C Thomas, Springfield, Illinois.

Imamura K, Ashida H, Ishikawa T, Fujii M. (1983) Human major psoas muscle and sacrospinalis muscle in relation to age: A study by computerised tomography. *J Gerontol*; **38**: 678–81.

Jacobs JM, Love S. (1985) Qualitative and quantitative morphology of human sural nerve at different ages. *Brain*; **108**: 897–924.

Lane WA. (1915) *The Operative Treatment of Chronic Intestinal Stasis*. James Nesbit, London

Larsson L. (1978) Morphological and functional characteristics of the ageing skeletal muscle in man: a cross sectional study. *Acta Physiol Scand* (Suppl); **458**: 1–36.

Larsson L. (1983) Histochemical characteristics of human skeletal muscle during aging. *Acta Physiol Scand*; **117**: 469–71.

Larsson L. (1982) Physical training effects on muscle morphology in sedentary males at different ages. *Med Sci Sports Exercise*; **14**: 203–6.

Lascelles RG, Thomas RK. (1966) Changes due to age in internodal length in the sural nerve in man. *J Neurol Neurosurg Psychiat*; **29**: 40–4.

Laurberg S, Swash M. (1989) Effects of aging on the anorectal sphincters and their innervation. *Dis Colon Rectum*; **32**: 737–42.

Lexell J, Henriksson-Larsen K, Winbald B, Sjostrom M. (1983) Distribution of different fibre types in human skeletal muscles; effects of ageing studied in whole muscle cross section. *Muscle and Nerve*; **6**: 588–95.

Loening-Baucke V, Anuras S. (1984a) Sigmoidal and rectal motility in healthy elderly subjects. *J Am Geriat Soc*; **32**: 887–91.

Loening-Baucke V, Anuras S. (1984b) Anorectal manometry in healthy elderly subjects. *J Am Geriat Soc*; **32**: 636–9.

Matheson DM, Keighley MRB. (1981) Manometric evaluation of rectal prolapse and faecal incontinence. *Gut*; **22**: 126–9.

McHugh SM, Diamant NE. (1987) Effect of age, gender, and parity on anal canal pressures. *Dig Dis Sci*; **32**: 726–36.

Milne JS, Williamson J. (1972) Bowel habit in older people. *Gerontol Clin*; **14**: 56–60.

Moore-Gillon V. (1984) Constipation: what does the patient mean? *J Roy Soc Med*; **77**: 108–10.

Neill ME, Swash M. (1980) Increased motor unit fibre density in the external anal sphincter in ano-rectal incontinence: a single fibre EMG study. *J Neurol Neurosurg Psychiat*; **43**: 343–7.

Ochoa J, Mair WGP. (1969) The normal sural nerve in man. 2. Changes in the axons and Schwann cells due to ageing. *Acta Neuropathol* (Berlin); **13**: 217–39.

Pearson MB, Bassey EJ, Bendall MJ. (1985) Muscle strength and anthropometric indices in elderly men and women. *Age and Ageing*; **14**: 49–54.

Percy JP, Neill ME, Kandiah TK, Swash M. (1982) A neurogenic factor in faecal incontinence in the elderly. *Age and Ageing*; **11**: 175–9.

Polgar J, Johnson MA, Weightman D, Appleton D. (1973) Data on the fiber size in thirty-six human muscles; an autopsy study. *J Neurol Sci*; **19**: 307–18.

Read NW, Harford WV, Schmulen AC, Read MG, Santa Ana CA, Fordtran JS. (1979) A clinical study of patients with faecal incontinence and diarrhoea. *Gastroenterology*; **76**: 747–56.

Read NW, Abouzekry L, Read MG, Howell P, Ottewell D, Donnelly TC. (1985) Anorectal function in elderly patients with faecal impaction. *Gastroenterology*. **89**: 959–66.

Read NW, Abouzekry L. (1986) Why do patients with faecal impaction have faecal incontinence? *Gut*; **27**: 283–7.

Rendtorff RC, Kashigarian M. (1966) Stool patterns of healthy adult males. *Dis Colon Rectum*; **10**: 222–8.

Rosenfalck P. (1975) *Electromyography–sensory and Motor Conductions: Findings in Normal Subjects*. Laboratory of Clinical Neurophysiology, Rikshozpitalet, Copenhagen. Cited in Swash M, Schwartz MS. (1981) *Neuromuscular Diseases, A Practical Approach to Diagnosis and Management*. Springer Verlag, Berlin.

Sica RGP, McComa AJ, Upton ARM, Longmire D. (1974) Motor unit estimations in small muscles of the hand. *J Neurol Neurosurg Psychiat*; **37**: 55–67.

Stalberg E, Thiele B. (1975) Motor unit fibre density in the extensor digitorum communis muscle. *J Neurol Neurosurg Psychiat*; **38**: 874–80.

Stalberg E, Trontelj JV. (1979) *Single Fibre Electromyography*. The Mirvalle Press Ltd, Old Woking, Surrey.

Swash M, Schwartz MS. (1981) *Neuromuscular Diseases, A Practical Approach to Diagnosis and Management*. Springer Verlag, Berlin.

Taylor PK. (1984) Non linear effects of age on nerve conduction in adults. *J Neurol Sci*; **66**: 223–34.

Tomlinson BE, Walton JN, Rebeiz JJ. (1969) The effects of ageing and cachexia upon skeletal muscle. A histopathological study. *J Neurol Sci*; **9**: 321–46.

Tomonaga M. (1977) Histochemical and ultrastructural changes in human skeletal muscle. *J Am Geriat Soc*; **25**: 125–31.

Wagman IH, Lesse H. (1952) Maximum conduction velocities of motor fibres of ulnar nerves in human subjects of various ages and sizes. *J Neurophysiol*; **15**: 235–44.

Wheatley IC, Hardy KJ, Dent J. (1977) Anal pressure studies in spinal patients. *Gut*; **18**: 488–90.

Yamagata A. (1965) Histopathological studies of the colon in relation to age. *Japan J Gastroenterol*; **62**; 229–35.

Young A, Stokes M, Crowe M. (1985) The size and strength of the quadriceps muscles of old and young men. *Clin Physiol*; **5**: 145–54.

8

Faecal incontinence in the elderly – introduction

The causes of faecal incontinence can be classified as:

1. Immobility
2. Symptomatic faecal incontinence
3. Faecal incontinence secondary to constipation and faecal impaction
4. Faecal incontinence secondary to cerebral disease:
   a) Impaired consciousness
   b) Patients with dementing illnesses
   c) Stroke
   d) Parkinson's Disease
5. Anorectal incontinence (idiopathic faecal incontinence)
   a) Anal sphincter and pelvic floor muscle weakness
   b) Anorectal sensory loss

Speakman and Kamm (1991) in a recent editorial recognised that faecal incontinence is the final disabling symptom of a number of heterogeneous anorectal abnormalities. This is particularly true in the elderly in whom the origin of faecal incontinence is usually multifactorial. The individual factors that contribute are listed above and are considered in Chapters 9–13, which will be followed by an overview of their relative contribution in Chapter 15. Chapters 11 and 12 are devoted to the discussion of the problem of constipation which is intimately related to faecal incontinence in the elderly.

Reference
Speakman CTM, Kamm MA. (1991) The internal anal sphincter – new insights into faecal incontinence. *Gut*; **32**: 345–6.

9

Anorectal function of elderly patients with faecal icontinence

Most of the studies on the anorectal function of patients with faecal incontinence have been performed on young and middle aged females. These patients, however, account for only a small proportion of the patients with faecal incontinence which is most prevalent among the elderly particularly those with other disabilities.

External anal sphincter function

The changes that occur in anorectal function with age were discussed on p. 61 with external anal sphincter weakness being the most prominent change. The anal squeeze pressure in the continent elderly has been found by Barrett et al. (1989) to be similar to that recorded using the same method and equipment in younger faecally incontinent patients ie. approximately 45cmH$_2$O (Kiff and Swash 1984).

Read and Abouzekry (1986) have suggested that the liability of elderly patients to develop faecal incontinence is increased by their age related anal sphincter weakness and that this is related to some degree of pudendal neuropathy. They quote a study performed by Percy et al. (1982) to support their conclusion.

Percy et al., (1982) performed single fibre EMG on six elderly patients with faecal incontinence and four continent elderly patients. They excluded patients with neurological disease or overt anorectal abnormalities from their study. The authors concluded that external sphincter fibre density was increased in their elderly incontinent patients. The study, however, is too small to allow any valid comparison of fibre density between the two groups and clearly does not produce direct evidence of pudendal neuropathy. Direct evidence of pudendal neuropathy occurring with increasing age is also lacking (see page 64) so although age related anal sphincter weakness may account for the high prevalence of faecal incontinence in the elderly, pudendal neuropathy cannot be implicated.

Anal squeeze pressures have been found to be similar in elderly faecally incontinent patients and elderly controls (see Fig. 23) (Barrett *et al.*, 1989). The presence of faecal incontinence is therefore not related to the degree of external sphincter weakness.

Pudendal nerve terminal motor latency is similar in elderly faecally incontinent and elderly control patients (Barrett *et al.*, 1989). Elderly patients with faecal incontinence differ therefore from younger incontinent patients in whom pudendal neuropathy is a prominent feature (Kiff and Swash, 1984; Snooks *et al.*, 1985) as it does not appear to be a major factor in the elderly.

The external sphincter response to rectal distension (inflation reflex) is absent in 61% of elderly faecally incontinent patients but this is not significantly different from elderly control patients 41% of whom also have an absent inflation reflex (Barrett *et al.*, 1989).

Internal anal sphincter dysfunction

The role of internal anal sphincter dysfunction as a cause of faecal incontinence in young and middle aged patients has been discussed in Chapter 6. It is also an important factor in elderly faecally incontinent patients. Barrett *et al.* (1989) demonstrated anal resting pressure to be significantly lower in these patients compared with elderly control patients and continent elderly faecally loaded patients (see Fig. 25).

Digital and manometric examination of the anus in these patients often reveals very low or undetectable anal tone. Rectal pressure in patients with gross faecal loading may therefore exceed anal pressure especially if the anus has previously been disrupted, e.g. surgically, when it may be seen to gape open.

Traditional geriatric medical teaching suggested that elderly faecally impacted patients become incontinent due to either stretch or reflex inhibition of the anal sphincter muscles (Tobin, 1987). There has never been any evidence to support this and evidence is now available to contradict this theory.

Barrett *et al.* (1989) found that anal resting pressures are similar in elderly patients with or without faecal loading and the recto-anal inhibitory reflex can still be elicited in faecally loaded patients. Read and Abouzekry (1986) have also shown that elderly patients with faecal impaction have similar anal pressures before and after disimpaction.

Some of the possible causes of internal sphincter weakness have been discussed in Chapter 6. The cause of internal sphincter weakness in the elderly is mostly unknown. It is possible that many elderly patients have internal sphincter weakness but retain continence until another event tips the balance towards incontinence, e.g. change of stool consistency to soft.

It is interesting to note that the onset of faeceal incontinence in diabetes

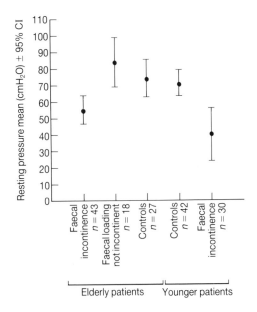

Fig. 25 Comparison of anal resting pressures (mean ± 95% confidence interval) between elderly and younger faecally incontinent patients and their controls. (Data from Barrett *et al.*, 1989)

tends to coincide with the onset of chronic diarrhoea (Schiller *et al.*, 1982). Internal sphincter dysfunction in these patients may be due to a defect in either the autonomic innervation or the smooth muscle. Diabetic autonomic neuropathy, however, does not invariably cause internal sphincter dysfunction as continent diabetic patients have normal resting pressure even though 79% have symptoms suggestive of autonomic neuropathy.

Other causes of autonomic degeneration may also affect continence. Studies of patients with progressive autonomic failure with multiple system atrophy have lead to the discovery of many interesting features of autonomic dysfunction (Mathias, 1987). Bladder dysfunction with frequency, urgency and urge incontinence is common in these patients (Kirkby and Bannister, 1986). They also exhibit low anal sphincter tone (Kirkby and Bannister, 1986) and faecal incontinence (Shy and Drager, 1960).

It is at present uncertain whether degeneration of the autonomic nervous system is a factor in faecal incontinence in the elderly.

Abnormalities in either the myenteric plexus or other components of the enteric nervous system could also influence the internal sphincter. The recto-anal inhibitory reflex can be considered to be a test of the integrity of the myenteric plexus. It is usually absent in patients with Hirschsprungs disease. Barrett *et al.*, (1989) were only able to elicit this reflex in 53% of their incontinent patients which was significantly less often than in their elderly control patients (82%). Read and Abouzekry (1986) in a similar study detected the reflex in 80% of their control group and in only 53% of their elderly impacted patients.

Hirschsprung's disease was not considered to be the cause of the absent reflex in these patients. It is likely, however, that myenteric plexus degeneration or damage is not the cause of the internal sphincter dysfunction identified in this study as normal internal sphincter pressures have been recorded in infants with Hirschsprung's disease (Howard and Nixon, 1968).

Further consideration is given later to the role of the myenteric plexus and the enteric nervous system in constipation (see p. 89).

Anal sensation

The effect of age on anal sensation has only been investigated in one study. Anal sensation appears to be impaired in the majority of elderly patients.

Barrett *et al.*, (1989) found that only 33% of their elderly control patients were able to discriminate between the presence of water and air instilled into the anal canal. A further 48% of their control patients however, correctly identified the presence of water in the anal canal. This impairment of anal sensation may possibly be due to a sensory neuropathy but they did not find any correlation between anal sensation and the pudendal nerve terminal motor latency.

The anal sensory abnormalities that are present in the elderly appear to contribute to their increased risk of faecal incontinence.

Anal sensation appears to be more severely impaired in incontinent geriatric patients as they were less aware of the presence of water or air in the anal canal than the control patients. Twenty five (57%) of the 46 incontinent geriatric patients assessed failed to identify either water or air instilled into the anal canal compared with just five (19%) of the 27 control patients assessed. Although cognitive impairment secondary to cerebral pathology, e.g. Alzheimers disease, may have contributed to this loss of awareness in incontinent patients, there does appear to be an abnormality in anal sensation similar to that reported in younger incontinent patients (Miller *et al.*, 1987; Roe *et al.*, 1986; Rogers *et al.*, 1988).

Loss of anal sensation as a single isolated factor, however, does not necessarily result in faecal incontinence, as Read and Read (1982) demonstrated that continence can be maintained when the anal canal is anaesthetised with lignocaine gel. This suggests that continence is only lost when a number of co-existent abnormalities are present.

Geriatric patients therefore have abnormalities in anal sensation, external sphincter strength and reflex activity which increase their risk of developing faecal incontinence. The main factor that appears to determine whether their continence is maintained is internal sphincter function.

Rectal sensation in faecal incontinence in the elderly

Abnormal rectal sensation does not appear to be a major factor in faecal incontinence. This will be discussed in Chapter 13.

References

Barrett JA, Brocklehurst JC, Kiff ES, Ferguson G, Faragher EB. (1989) Anal function in geriatric patients with faecal incontinence. *Gut*; **30**: 1244–51.

Howard ER, Nixon HH. (1968) Internal anal sphincter. Observations on development and mechanisms of inhibitory responses in premature infants and children with Hirschsprung's disease. *Arch Dis Childhood*; **43**: 569–578.

Kiff ES, Swash M. (1984) Slowed conduction in the pudendal nerves in idiopathic (neurogenic) faecal incontinence. *Br J Surg*; **71**: 614–16.

Kirkby RS, Bannister R. (1986) Bladder dysfunction in progressive autonomic failure. *Br Med J*. **293**: 223–4.

Mathias CJ. (1987) Autonomic dysfunction. *Br J Hosp Med*; **38**: 238–43.

Miller R, Bartolo DCC, Cervero F, Mortensen NJMcC. (1987) Anorectal temperature sensation: a comparison of normal and incontinent patients. *Br J Surg*; **74**: 511–15.

Percy JP, Neill ME, Kandiah TK, Swash M. (1982) A neurogenic factor in faecal incontinence in the elderly. *Age and Ageing*. **11**: 175–9.

Read MG, Read NW. (1982) Role of anorectal sensation in preserving continence. *Gut*; **23**: 345–7.

Read NW, Abouzekry L. (1986) Why do patients with faecal impaction have faecal incontinence. *Gut*; **27**: 283–7.

Roe AM, Bartolo DCC, Mortensen NJMcC. (1986) New method for assessment of anal sensation in various anorectal disorders. *Br J Surg*; **73**: 310–12.

Rogers J, Henry MM, Misiewicz JJ. (1988) Combined sensory and motor deficit in primary neuropathic faecal incontinence. *Gut*; **29**: 5–9.

Schiller LR, Santa Ana CA, Schmulen AC, Hendler RS, Harford WV, Fordtran JS. (1982) Pathogenesis of fecal incontinence in diabetes mellitus. Evidence for internal anal sphincter dysfunction. *New Eng J Med*; **307**: 1666–71.

Shy GM, Drager GA. (1960) A neurological syndrome associated with orthostatic hypotension. *Arch Neurol*; **2**: 511–27.

Snooks SJ, Henry MM, Swash M. (1985) Anorectal incontinence and rectal prolapse: differential assessment of the innervation to puborectalis and external anal sphincter muscles. *Gut*; **26**: 470–6.

Tobin GW. (1987) Incontinence in the elderly. *Practitioner*; **231**: 843–7.

10

Symptomatic faecal incontinence and its management

Faecal incontinence may be the presenting feature of colorectal disease especially if it is associated with diarrhoea. The following causes should always be considered in the elderly: infective diarrhoea; carcinoma of the rectum or colon; proctitis or colitis (due to either ischaemiaor, inflammatory bowel disease); diverticular disease; drugs, especially laxatives; malabsorption syndromes and other causes of chronic diarrhoea.

Faecal incontinence due to one of these causes should be treated by treating the underlying disease. The more common problems are reviewed below.

Colorectal tumours

The incidence of lower gastrointestinal tumours (adenoma or carcinoma) increases with age. The typical presentation is with a change of bowel habit, rectal bleeding, weight loss or large bowel obstruction. Some patients may present with incontinence. The diagnosis therefore needs to be considered in faecally incontinent patients especially when other suggestive symptoms and signs are present. These patients require prompt examination of the lower gastrointestinal tract starting with digital rectal examination which is traditionally followed, in the presence of rectal bleeding, by sigmoidoscopy and double contrast barium enema and then colonoscopy if the other investigations were negative.

The use of these investigations has recently been re-assessed as Wolf *et al.* (1986) demonstrated that elderly and/or debilitated patients are often not capable of manoeuvring well enough on an X-ray table to give high quality barium studies. Negative results from unsatisfactory studies may not therefore exclude the presence of disease and the examination may be a very unpleasant experience.

The preparation required for a barium enema should be considered carefully when requesting this examination as many elderly patients experience faecal incontinence following administration of the potent laxatives used in the preparation. Elderly people with disabilities therefore should be admitted to hospital when they are having the bowel preparation unless they have a competent carer who can ensure that the patient has a sufficient fluid intake and does not suffer any other adverse effects of the preparation, e.g. dehydration or hypotension

Comparative studies of colonoscopy versus barium enema in the investigation of possible colonic adenoma, carcinoma or angiodysplasia have concluded that colonoscopy is the investigation of choice in the elderly as it is more sensitive than barium enema (Irvine *et al.*, 1988; Rex *et al.*, 1990). The comparative rate of complications in the elderly, however, has not been assessed.

Detection of a colonic or rectal carcinoma should be followed by a surgical assessment. The surgeon may, however, be faced with a major dilemma about whether to remove a resectable lesion if the patient is very old as old age has been used for many years as an excuse not to operate. Recent studies however indicate that although there is a higher mortality in large bowel cancer surgery in the elderly (12% vs 3%) (Fielding *et al.*, 1989) this is almost entirely due to the increased risk associated with emergency surgery compared to routine surgery. Pre-operative assessment of high risk patients may, however, help to reduce the risks (Seymour and Vaz, 1987) as more than half of the deaths are due to cardiopulmonary complications. Palliative local treatment, e.g. laser therapy, is now available as an alternative (Barr *et al.*, 1989; Krasner, 1989).

The prognosis of colorectal cancer in the elderly has been found to be similar to that of younger patients (Irvin, 1988). Many elderly patients unfortunately present too late for curative surgery and consequently only palliative surgery is possible which is associated with a high mortality rate due to the presence of widespread local and/or distant disease (Lewis and Khoury, 1988).

Much effort has therefore been directed towards the early detection of tumours. The Nottingham trial of faecal occult blood testing as a screening test for asymptomatic large bowel cancer has detected approximately two carcinomas per 1000 people screened (Thomas *et al.*, 1990). The effect that the screening programme has on mortality from the disease is awaited.

The occult blood screening tests have recently been the subject of some investigation. None was found to be perfect. The best sensitivity recorded in Pye *et al.*'s (1990) series was 54% for the Haemoccult test. Tate *et al.* (1990) suggest therefore that a negative Haemoccult test does not exclude colonic blood loss and should not therefore be used to influence symptomatic patients' management.

Compliance with screening for occult blood loss is more likely to be achieved with three day testing compared with more prolonged tests with no significant loss of sensitivity in symptomatic patients (Thomas *et al.*, 1990).

Infective diarrhoea

Infective causes of diarrhoea account for many acute cases of faecal incontinence especially in debilitated old people who are rendered immobile and perhaps confined to bed by their acute illness. Two of the most common infecting organisms are the Salmonella and Campylobacter species. They may cause enterocolitis which is potentially fatal in debilitated old people. Pseudomembranous colitis secondary to *Clostridium difficile* infection should also be considered especially when diarrhoea occurs either during or after a course of antibiotic treatment.

Salmonella

Salmonellosis is the commonest cause of food poisoning in England and Wales. During the 1980s the incidence steadily increased. The worst outbreak of salmonella food poisoning during that period was at the Stanley Royd Hospital. This affected 400 patients and staff and resulted in the death of 19 elderly patients.

In the early 1980s the increase was mainly due to *Salmonella typhimurium* infections but since 1985 there has been a dramatic increase in the occurence of *Salmonella enteritidis* infection (Sharp, 1988). *Salmonella enteritidis* phage type 4 has emerged as an important cause and occurs sporadically in 90% of cases (Cowden *et al.*, 1989). Eggs, egg products and precooked chickens are recognised as important vehicles for infection with *S. enteritidis* phage type 4. This is considered to be very important because 30 million eggs are consumed daily in the United Kingdom which represents a major public health problem despite the low rates of infection among the poultry flocks.

Public health initiatives have lead to attempts to eradicate *S. enteritidis* from poultry flocks, to discourage the consumption of raw eggs and to improve hygiene standards in kitchens.

Most cases of enterocolitis caused by salmonella species resolve quickly and without complications with simple symptomatic treatment. The most important component of which is adequate fluid and electrolyte replacement. Antibiotics are not indicated for routine use but are indicated when there is evidence of systemic spread, e.g. enteric fever or impaired host resistance to infection. Chloramphenicol is the antibiotic of choice in most areas of the world but ampicillin and third generation cephalosporins, e.g. cefotaxime and ciprofloxacin, are also active.

Campylobacter

Campylobacter colitis is a common cause of severe bloody diarrhoea which may be mistaken for ulcerative colitis and is usually due to *Campylobacter jejuni* infection. Patients are often severely dehydrated and require fluid and electrolyte replacement. Unlike Salmonella infections, treatment with antibiotics does not prolong the carriage of *C. jejuni*. Erythromycin, which is the treatment of choice, eliminates carriage within 72 hours in most patients (Anders *et al.*, 1982).

Inflammatory bowel disease

The inflammatory bowel diseases ulcerative colitis and Crohn's disease occasionally present with faecal incontinence in old age.

Ulcerative Colitis

The presentation of ulcerative colitis in the elderly is similar to that in younger subjects. with diarrhoea (100%), rectal bleeding (58%), abdominal pain (41%) and weight loss (30%) being the commonest symptoms (Gupta *et al.*, 1985). It has been suggested that rectal bleeding may be less common and weight loss more common in the elderly (Zimmerman *et al.*, 1985).

The commonest pattern of disease activity is a proctitis or disease limited to the left side of the colon rather than a pancolitis. Substantial colitis, i.e. disease extending proximal to the splenic flexure, is present in approximately 23% of elderly patients (Gupta *et al.*, 1985; Jones and Hoare, 1988).

Active disease is often associated with anaemia, neutrophilia, raised ESR and hypoalbuminaemia. The onset of the disease or its subsequent relapse exhibits seasonal variation but no factors have been found to be significantly associated with disease relapse (Riley *et al.*, 1990)

The diagnosis of ulcerative colitis is based on histological evidence of the disease in a rectal biopsy taken during a careful sigmoidoscopy after the exclusion of infective causes of colitis. Barium enema and / or colonoscopy may outline diffuse abnormalities extending proximally from the rectum to confirm the diagnosis and allow the extent of the disease to be determined. Many patients have extra-intestinal manifestations of the disease which may include joint, ocular, skin and liver complications.

Ulcerative colitis patients have increased levels of colonic substance P (Goldin *et al.*, 1989).

The anorectal function of ulcerative colitis patients has been studied by Rao *et al.*, (1988). Their patients were categorised at the time of the study to be either in the active phase of the disease or to be quiescent. They were compared with normal controls. Anal manometry studies were found to be normal. Resting rectal activity was found to be reduced in active colitics in whom rectal contractions were recorded for only 12% of the total recording time, compared with 37% for similar studies in quiescent colitics or controls.

Rectal saline infusion tests revealed that the volume of saline infused into the rectum before leakage occurred was significantly lower in colitic patients irrespective of activity compared to control patients. Saline infusion induced regular rectal contractions in all the subjects studied. In 67% of the continent active colitics the peaks of rectal pressure exceeded the anal relaxation pressures that coincided with the rectal contractions. Peak rectal pressure exceeded anal relaxation pressure throughout the study in the incontinent colitics.

The amplitude of the rectal contractions is greater in active colitics than in the quiescent patients and controls which suggests that the colitic rectum is hyperactive (Rao et al., 1987b, Reddy et al., 1991). Reddy et al. (1991) also demonstrated that the pressure is uniform throughout the colon unlike the pressure gradient observed in normal individuals (see p. 32).

The transit of radio-opaque markers has been found to be rapid through the sigmoid colon and rectum which would account for colitic patients voiding small stools frequently (Rao et al., 1987a). The frequency of propagating colonic contractions is higher in these patients than in normal subjects though the amplitude is reduced (Reddy et al., 1991). Scintigraphy studies have shown that transit is variable in the colon in these patients (Reddy et al., 1991). The same group have produced similar results in patients with functional diarrhoea (Bazzocchi et al., 1991).

The inability of the active colitics to retain even small volumes of saline infused into the rectum would account for the inability of many of these patients to retain steroid enemas (Ruddell et al., 1980).

The medical treatment of ulcerative colitis is not affected by the age of the patient. Steroids are used in the treatment of acute severe episodes. In less severe cases sulphasalazine may be used to induce remission and is also used for maintenance treatment.

Recent developments in treatment have been reviewed by Hawkey and Hawthorne (1988). The 5 aminosalicylic acid (5-ASA) component of sulphasalazine has been found to be as effective at inducing and maintaining remission as sulphasalazine (Riley et al., 1988a). It is available commercially as Mesalazine and Olsalazine and appears to be particularly valuable for patients who are intolerant of sulphasalazine (Riley et al., 1988b, Meyers et al., 1987, Rao et al., 1989). In addition potential for further development may be possible because higher concentrations of 5-ASA can be delivered to the colon than would be tolerable when combined with the sulphapyridine component. Topical preparations of salicylate are now available and are of particular use for those with proctosigmoiditis or poorly responsive proctitis.

Hayllar and Bjarnason (1991) suggest that sulphasalazine should not be discarded as an outmoded treatment in favour of the more modern 5-ASA compounds until there is greater understanding of the ways in which these drugs work, as serious renal side effects have been reported with Mesalazine (CSM, 1990). Some of the beneficial effects of sulphasalazine on the inflammatory process may be due to the combination rather than just 5- ASA alone.

Kiilerich et al., (1992), in a comparative study of Olsalazine versus sulphasalazine on 227 patients, found that 7% of patients had adverse drug reactions. There was no significant difference between the drugs in this or in the relapse rate during 12 months' treatment.

Steroids remain the main acute therapy for severe exacerbations of ulcerative colitis despite the potential for side effects in the elderly. A new appreciation of their use in maintenance may be possible with the development of poorly absorbed oral steroids with topical activity in the colon. Topical preparations of steroids for rectal installation are valuable for proctosigmoiditis. Some elderly people, however, have difficulty with these. The frequency with which proctosigmoiditis appears in the elderly suggests that trials of such preparations in this age group are important.

Elderly patients with ulcerative colitis appear to have higher surgical fatality rates (Ritchie *et al.*, 1984) than younger patients but their overall mortality does not appear to be increased. Gupta *et al.* (1985) found that all 17 patients over the age of 65 years included in their study responded well to medical management. Only five patients had recurrent attacks and none required surgery. Jones and Hoare (1988) compared 43 patients aged over 65 years at diagnosis with 124 patients diagnosed before the age of 55 years. They found no significant difference between the two groups with regard to symptom free years or number of hospital admissions. No patient required – emergency surgery and only two (5%) required elective surgery for persistent ill health. The cumulative incidence of surgery in patients of all ages has been recorded as 2% at five years and 15% at ten years. The higher surgical fatality rate in the elderly may be due to emergency surgery being performed for the complications of severe ulcerative colitis e.g. perforation or toxic dilation of the colon rather than less urgent surgery for persistent disease.

More information is still required about the natural history of ulcerative colitis in the elderly with attention being concentrated on patients with distal colitis and proctitis, as previous studies have concentrated on patients with either severe disease or requiring surgery. Questions about the timing and type of surgery in elderly patients still need to be answered. A recent review has suggested old age (> 60 years) to be a possible contra-indication to this operation (Kumar and Williams, 1990) but this view is controversial.

In the past the surgical treatment was total proctocolectomy with an ileostomy but now the treatment of choice is the cosmetically more acceptable restorative proctocolectomy with the fashioning of an ileal pouch which is anastomosed to the anus with the aim being to preserve or restore continence. This, however, is not always successful.

The best method of fashioning the ileo-anal anastomosis is still under investigation (Keighley *et al.*, 1988; Holdsworth and Johnston, 1988; Phillips, 1991). It has been suggested (Miller *et al.*, 1990a) that preservation of anal sensation by retaining the anal mucosa will reduce the incidence of incontinence post-operatively but this requires longer follow-up to determine the effects upon continence as well as determining the risks of local recurrence of the disease. Miller *et al.* (1990b) found ileo-anal pouch activity to be usually quiescent with very little sampling activity. The one patient in their study with frequent pouch contraction was regularly incontinent of faeces.

Crohn's Disease

Crohn's disease occurring in later life is less common than ulcerative colitis but the overall incidence is steadily increasing. Colonic involvement is more common in the elderly (40%) than in younger patients (6%) but the distal ileum is still the commonest site of disease (55%) in elderly patients presenting with Crohn's disease (Fabricus *et al.*, 1985). Extensive colonic or small bowel disease is uncommon in the elderly.

Elderly patients with Crohn's disease present in a fashion similar to their younger counterparts. Diarrhoea (often mild) (100%), weight loss (57%), abdominal pain (29%) and rectal bleeding (29%) are the most common symptoms of Crohn's disease (Gupta *et al.*, 1985).

Physical examination may reveal an abdominal mass or anorectal disease such as fissures, skin tags, fistulae or perianal abscess. As in ulcerative colitis, non-specific features such as anaemia, raised ESR and hypoalbuminaemia may be found and malabsorption may occur if small bowel is also involved.

The diagnosis usually depends upon the typical radiological features being identified on small bowel meal and/or barium enema, i.e. deep ulcers producing a cobblestone effect, skip lesions due to the non-diffuse nature of the disease, and fistulae.

Endoscopy may also be helpful especially when there is colonic or rectal involvement. The typical endoscopic and biopsy appearance of Crohn's disease is granulomatous change. Difficult diagnostic problems may occur in differentiating Crohn's disease from the far more common conditions of colonic neoplasm or diverticulosis, especially as these may co-exist. Ischaemic change in the bowel may also produce diagnostic difficulty as segmental involvement may occur (Brandt *et al.*, 1981).

The medical management of Crohn's disease is not affected by age though more attention may need to be given to nutritional and vitamin status in the elderly.

The role of salazopyrine or its derivatives in the management of Crohn's disease is not as clear as in ulcerative colitis, especially as a prophylactic agent. It does appear to be effective in the treatment of colonic Crohn's disease and may therefore be especially useful for elderly Crohn's patients. Acute episodes of Crohn's disease should be managed with steroids. Metronidazole is useful in patients with anorectal complications (Ursing *et al.*, 1982).

Immunosuppresive drugs, e.g. azathioprine and 6-mercaptopurine, are valuable in patients who do not respond to either steroids or metronidazole and in patients on high dose steroids in whom it is difficult to reduce the dose. The use of these drugs has not been specifically studied in elderly patients and their position in treatment regimens is not yet clear.

Elderly patients seem to have a standardised mortality ratio very similar to the average for Crohn's disease patients of all ages, which is usually quoted as twice that of the general population (Prior *et al.*, 1981).

The course of the disease seems to depend very much on the anatomical site of the disease. A Birmingham study has reported that most patients in whom distal ileitis predominates require laparotomy at some time during the course of their disease either to make the diagnosis or for obstructive symptoms or perforation. Frequently this was early in the course of their illness, following which most remained well with medical management (Fabricus *et al.*, 1985). Patients in whom colonic disease predominates and who receive medical management tend to require fewer surgical interventions (23%) compared with a 39% accumulated probability of bowel surgery at ten years (Elliot *et al.*, 1985).

Further information is still required about late onset Crohn's disease, particularly on the course and prognosis of Crohn's colitis and proctitis and late recurrence of the disease after surgical procedures in the elderly.

Bile acid diarrhoea

Malabsorption of bile acids may be an important factor in the patho-genesis of diarrhoea (Merrick *et al.*, 1985; Mitchell *et al.*, 1973) and may also be an aetiological factor in some patients with the irritable bowel syndrome (Merrick *et al.*, 1985).

Edwards *et al.*, (1989) infused deoxycholic acid into the rectum of 11 healthy volunteers and found that even low concentrations increased rectal sensitivity, reducing the distension volume required to pro-duce a desire to defaecate. Higher concentrations produced extreme rectal discomfort and urgency which was associated with large rectal contractions.

References

Anders BJ, Lauer BA, Paisley JW, Reller LB. (1982) Double blind placebo con-trolled trial of erythromycin in the treatment of *Campylobacter enteritis*. *Lancet*; i: 131–2.

Barr H, Bown SG, Krasner N, Boulos PB. (1989) Photodynamic therapy for colorectal disease. *Int J Colorect Dis*; **4**: 15–19.

Bazzocchi G, Ellis J, Villanueva-Meyer J, Reddy SN, Mena I, Snape WJ. (1991) Effect of eating on colonic motility and transit in patients with functional diarrhoea. *Gastroenterology*; **101**: 1298–1306.

Brandt LJ, Boley SJ, Goldberg L, Mitsudo S, Berman A. (1981) Colitis in the elderly: a reappraisal. *Am J Gastroenterol*; **76**: 239–45.

Committee on Safety of Medicines. (1990) Current Problems. December.

Cowden JM, Lynch D, Joseph CA, O'Mahony M, Mawer SL, Rowe B, Bartlett CLR. (1989) Case-control study of infections with Salmonella enteritidis phage type 4 in England. British Medical Journal. 299: 771–773.

Edwards CA, Brown S, Baxter AJ, Bannister JJ, Read NW. (1989) Effect of bile acid on anorectal function in man. *Gut*. **30**: 383–6.

Elliott PR, Ritchie JK, Lennard-Jones JE. (1985) Prognosis of colonic Crohn's disease. *Br Med J*; **291**: 178.

Fabricus PJ, Gyde SN, Shouler P, Keighley MRB, Alexander-Williams J, Allan RN. (1985) Crohn's disease in the elderly. *Gut*; **26**: 461–5.

Fielding LP, Phillips RKS, Hittinger R. (1989) Factors influencing mortality after curative surgery for large bowel cancer in elderly patients. *Lancet*; i: 595–7.

Goldin E, Karmeli F, Selinger Z, Rachmilewitz D. (1989) Colonic substance P levels are increased in ulcerative colitis and decreased in chronic severe constipation. *Dig Dis Sci*; **34**: 754–7.

Gupta S, Saverymuttu SH, Keshavarzian A, Hodgson HJF. (1985) Is the pattern of inflammatory bowel disease different in the elderly? *Age and Ageing*; **14**: 366–70.

Hawkey CJ, Hawthorne AB. (1988) Medical treatment of ulcerative colitis: scoring the advances. *Gut*; **29**: 1298–1303.

Hayllar J, Bjarnason IB. (1991) Sulphasalazine in ulcerative colitis: in memoriam? *Gut*; **32**: 462–3.

Holdsworth PJ, Johnston D. (1988) Anal sensation after restorative proctocolectomy for ulcerative colitis. *Br J Surg*; **75**: 993–6.

Irvin TT. (1988) Prognosis of colorectal cancer in the elderly. *Br J Surg*; **75**: 419–21.

Irvine EJ, O'Connor, Frost RA, *et al*. (1988) Prospective comparison of double contrast barium enema plus flexible sigmoidoscopy *v*. colonoscopy in rectal bleeding: barium enema *v*. colonoscopy in rectal bleeding. *Gut*; **29**: 1188–93.

Jones HW, Hoare AM. (1988) Does ulcerative colitis behave differently in the elderly? *Age and Ageing*; **17**: 410–14.

Keighley MRB, Yoshioka K, Kmiot W, Heyen F. (1988) Physiological parameters influencing function in restorative proctocolectomy and ileo- pouch-anal anastomosis. *Br J Surg*; **75**: 997–1002.

Kiilerich S, Ladefoged K, Rannem T, Ranlov PJ and the Danish Olsalazine Study Group. (1992) Prophylactic effects of Olsalazine *v*. sulphasalazine during 12 months maintenance treatment of ulcerative colitis. *Gut*. **33**: 252–3.

Krasner N. (1989) Laser therapy in the management of benign and malignant tumours in the colon and rectum. *Int J Colorect Dis*; **4**: 2–5.

Kumar D, Williams NS. (1990) Surgical management of ulcerative colitis. *Hosp Update*; **16**: 113–20.

Lewis AAM, Khoury GA. (1988) Resection for colorectal cancer in the very old: are the risks too high? *Br Med J*; **296**: 459–61.

Merrick MV, Eastwood MA, Ford MJ. (1985) Is bile acid malabsorption underdiagnosed? An evaluation of accuracy of diagnosis by measurement of ScHCAT retention. *Br Med J*; **290**: 665–8.

Meyers S, Sacher DB, Present DH, Janowitz B. (1987) Olsalazine sodium in the treatment of ulcerative colitis among patients intolerant of sulphasalazine. A prospective, randomised, placebo controlled, double blind, dose ranging trial. *Gastroenterology*; **93**: 1255–62.

Miller R, Bartolo DCC, Orrom WJ, Mortensen NJMcC, Roe AM, Cervero F. (1990a) Improvement of anal sensation with preservation of the anal transition zone after ileoanal anastomosis for ulcerative colitis. *Dis Colon Rectum*; **33**: 414–18.

Miller R, Orrom WJ, Duthie G, Bartolo DCC, Mortensen NJMcC. (1990b) Ambulatory anorectal physiology in patients following restorative proctocolectomy for ulcerative colitis: comparison with normal controls. *Br J Surg*; **77**: 895–7.

Mitchell WD, Findlay JM, Prescott RJ, Eastwood MA, Horn DB. (1973) Bile acids in the diarrhoea of ileal resection. *Gut*; **14**: 348–53.

Phillips RKS. (1991) Pelvic pouches. *Br J Surg*; **78**: 1025–6.

Prior P, Gyde S, Cooke WT, Waterhouse JAH, Allan RN. (1981) Mortality in Crohn's disease. *Gastroenterology*; **80**: 307–12.

Pye G, Jackson J, Thomas WM, Hardcastle JD. (1990) Comparison of Coloscreen Self-Test and Haemoccult faecal occult blood tests in the detection of colorectal cancer in symptomatic patients. *Br J Surg*; **77**: 630–1.

Rao SC, Read NW, Davison PA, Bannister JJ, Holdsworth CD. (1987b) Anorectal sensitivity and responses to rectal distension in patients with ulcerative colitis. *Gastroenterology*; **93**: 1270–5.

Rao SC, Read NW, Brown C, Bruce C, Holdsworth CD. (1987a) Studies on the mechanism of bowel disturbance in ulcerative colitis. *Gastroenterology*; **93**: 1013–19.

Rao SC, Read NW, Stobart JAH, Haynes WG, Benjamin S, Holdsworth CD. (1988) Anorectal contractility under basal conditions and during rectal infusion of saline in ulcerative colitis. *Gut*; **29**: 769–77.

Rao SC, Dundas SAC, Holdsworth CD, Cann PA, Palmer KR, Corbett CL. (1989) Olsalazine or sulphasalazine in first attacks of ulcerative colitis? A double blind study. *Gut*; **30**: 675–9.

Reddy SN, Bazzocchi G, Chan S, et al. (1991) Colonic motility and transit in health and Ulcerative colitis. *Gastroenterology*; **101**: 1289–97.

Rex DK, Weddle RA, Lehman GA, et al. (1990) Flexible sigmoidoscopy plus air contrast barium enema versus colonoscopy for suspected lower gastrointestinal bleeding. *Gastroenterology*; **98**: 855–61.

Riley SA, Mani V, Goodman MJ, Herd ME, Dutt S, Turnberg LA. (1988a) Comparison of delayed release 5-aminosalicylic acid (Mesalazine) and sulfasalazine in the treatment of mild to moderate ulcerative colitis relapse. *Gut*; **29**: 669–74.

Riley SA, Mani V, Goodman MJ, Herd ME, Dutt S, Turnberg LA. (1988b) Comparison of delayed release 5-aminosalicylic acid (Mesalazine) and sulfasalazine as maintenance treatment for patients with ulcerative colitis. *Gastroenterology*; **94**: 1383–9.

Riley SA, Mani V, Goodman MJ, Lucas S. (1990) Why do patients with ulcerative colitis relapse? *Gut*; **31**: 179–83.

Ritchie JK, Ritchie SM, McIntyre PB, Marks CG. (1984) Management of acute severe ulcerative colitis in district hospitals. *J Roy Soc Med*; **77**: 465–71.

Ruddell WSJ, Dickinson RJ, Dixon MF, Axon ATR. (1980) Treatment of distal ulcerative colitis in relapse: comparison of hydrocortisone enemas and rectal hydrocortisone foam. *Gut*; **21**: 885–9.

Seymour DG, Vaz FG. (1987) Aspects of surgery in the elderly: preoperative medical assessment. *Br J Hosp Med*; **37**: 431–5.

Sharp JCM. (1988) Salmonellosis and eggs. *Br Med J*; **297**: 1557–8

Tate JJT, Northway J, Royle GT, Taylor I. (1990) Faecal occult blood testing in symptomatic patients: comparison of three tests. *Br J Surg*; **77**: 523–6.

Thomas WM, Pye G, Hardcastle JD, Mangham CM. (1990) Faeceal occult blood screening for colorectal neoplasms: a randomised trial of three days or six days of tests. *Br J Surg*; **77**: 277–9.

Ursing B, Alm T, Barany F. et al. (1982) A comparative study of metranidazole and sulfasalazine for active Crohn's disease. The cooperative Crohn's disease study in Sweden. II: Result. *Gastroenterology*; **83**: 550–62.

Wolf EL, Frager D, Beneventano T. (1986) Feasibility of double contrast barium enema in the elderly. *Am J Radiol*; **145**: 47–8.

Zimmerman J, Gavish D, Rachmilewitz D. (1985) Early and late onset ulcerative colitis. Distinct clinical features. *J Clin Gastroenterol*; **7**: 492–8.

11

Idiopathic constipation

The term 'constipation' is is usually used to indicate either infrequent defaecation (less than three stools passed per week) or excessive straining on defaecation. The main recognised causes of defaecatory difficulty are hard stool and obstructed defaecation. Constipation may be the presenting symptom of underlying colonic disease, among which carcinoma of the colon must always be considered, especially in the elderly. The common diseases which may cause constipation are listed in Table 1.

The main features of idiopathic constipation include slow intestinal transit, abnormal defaecation and impaired rectal sensation. Constipated patients stools are usually hard and are often small pellets or scybala. There are, however, exceptions to this which are discussed further in Chapter 12.

Colonic motility/transit

Constipated patients can be divided on the basis of their whole gut transit times into slow transit or normal transit constipation (Preston 1985). Delayed transit tends to occur mainly in the colon and/or the rectum.

The first research studies performed on constipated patients employed a variety of techniques to assess colonic motility but the emphasis has now shifted to the assessment of transit as pressure changes in the lumen of the gut are less relevant than their effects, i.e. colonic transit.

Patients with idiopathic constipation are a heterogeneous group who exhibit a variety of abnormalities of colonic transit (Chaussade *et al.*, 1989;, Kamm *et al.*, 1988) and colonic motility (Meunier *et al.*, 1979;

Lanfranchi *et al.*, 1984; Preston and Lennard-Jones 1985a; Bazzocchi *et al.*, 1990).

Chaussade *et al.*, (1989) performed segmental colonic transit studies on 91 constipated patients using the method described by Metcalf *et al.*, (1987). Their patients ingested 20 radio-opaque pellets on days 1, 2 and 3. Abdominal radiographs were taken on days 4 and 7 at the same time of day as the pellets were ingested. Further radiographs were performed on day 10 on the patients who still had pellets present on the day 7 radiograph. The projection zones of the right colon, left colon and rectosigmoid were identified and used in the calculation of the segmental transit time. Four types of colonic transit response were found: normal colonic transit (54%); right colonic stasis (18%); outlet obstruction (13%); and isolated left colonic stasis (15%).

Meunier *et al.* (1979) found that two-thirds of their group of constipated patients (mean age 40 years) had normal sigmoid colonic motility with the remaining patients being equally divided between hypomotility and hypermotility states.

Lanfranchi *et al.* (1984) compared constipated patients suffering pain with painless constipation patients. They found that their transit times to the caecum were similar though patients with painless constipation

Table 1 Causes of constipation

General factors	Immobility
	Dehydration
	Inadequate diet
	Anorectal abnormalities
Drugs	Opiates
	Anticholinergic agents
	Antidepressants
	Diuretics
	Aluminium containing antacids
	Laxatives
Gut lesions	Intestinal obstruction – carcinoma
	– other causes
	Aganglionosis – Hirschsprung's disease
	– laxative induced
	Idiopathic megacolon
Neurological	Paraplegia
	Stroke
	Parkinson's disease
	Multiple sclerosis
Endocrine	Panhypopituitarism
	Hyperparathyroidism
Psychiatric	Depression
	Dementia
Metabolic	Hypercalcaemia
	Hypokalaemia

had prolonged whole gut transit time due to delay in the colon. They suggested that painful constipation was synonymous with the irritable colon.

Dynamic colonic scintigraphy has enabled assessment of colonic transit to be performed (see p. 30). Patients with severe idiopathic constipation exhibit a spectrum of colonic abnormalities ranging from slow transit involving only the rectum and sigmoid colon to slow transit involving the whole colon. Kamm *et al.* (1988) found that the transit time from the hepatic flexure to the rectum for the 'head of the isotope column' in normals ranged from 1–10 minutes (mean 5.3 minutes) whereas the corresponding time in four constipated patients was 14–25 minutes. In their three other patients the radio-isotope failed to reach the rectum in two hours. The patients also showed relatively impaired transport of the isotope 'mass'.

Kamm *et al.* (1988) also found that the arrival of the isotope in the rectum resulted in a strong desire to defaecate with subsequent elimination of 69–97% of the radioactivity in a single stool in normal individuals. The corresponding proportion of the total isotope excreted by the four patients was 50%, 59%, 77% and 86%. The other three patients in whom the isotope front did not reach the rectum during the two hour imaging period did not experience a call to stool and did not defaecate whilst undergoing the study. Abdominal cramps were experienced by all the normal individuals but not by any of the patients in whom no transit occurred.

Colonic faecal loading was not the cause of the transit delay in the patients studied as measures were taken to ensure that the colon was clear before the studies were performed.

In another scintigraphic study Stivland *et al.* (1991) examined eight patients with idiopathic constipation who had normal ability to defaecate. Patients in this study swallowed radiolabelled resin particles to allow measurement of gastric emptying, small bowel transit and colonic transit once the particles disintegrated in the colon. Seven of the eight patients had slow colonic transit due to either exaggerated reservoir function of the ascending and transverse colon and/or impaired propulsive activity in the descending colon.

Although patients with idiopathic constipation demonstrate differing patterns of colonic motility they are consistent in their lack of colonic propulsive activity in response to eating (Bazzocchi *et al.*, 1990) and in having a significant reduction in colonic mass movements (Bassotti *et al.*, 1988).

Electrical activity

The control mechanism for normal colonic motility is complex and poorly understood compared with the control of small bowel motility and its abnormalities which are better understood. Smooth muscle cell membrane electrical activity, intrinsic and extrinsic nervous activity and hormonal activity all appear to play a role (Huizinga and Daniel, 1986). Electrical activity recorded from the colon is recognised to be different from that recorded in the stomach and small bowel.

Colonic myoelectric spiking activity was assessed by Dapoigny *et al.* (1988) using ring electrodes mounted at 5cm intervals on a 0.5cm diameter PVC tube positioned in the colon using a colonoscope. They found two types of activity: short spike bursts lasting approximately four seconds only on one electrode at any one time and long spike bursts lasting approximately 20–30 seconds. The long spike bursts were sometimes propagated.

Long spike bursts were seen more frequently in the left colon than right colon before the test meal. After the meal there was an increase in long spike burst activity throughout the colon which was more marked in the left colon, especially the rectosigmoid, than the right colon. Short spike burst activity was unaltered by the test meal.

Nervous control of colonic transit

The cause of the slow colonic transit has been investigated by assessing its nervous control.

Preston and Lennard-Jones (1985a) recognised that slow transit constipation may be due to a myenteric plexus abnormality as degeneration of the plexus was found in colectomy specimens excised from patients with intractable chronic constipation (Preston *et al.*, 1983b, Krishnamurphy *et al.*, 1985). They therefore instilled the stimulant laxative bisacodyl, which acts on the myenteric plexus (Hardcastle and Mann 1968), into the colon of patients with slow transit constipation and found that this produced progressive peristaltic waves in 11 (61%) patients. The remaining seven patients (39%) did not respond, which was thought to indicate a possible myenteric plexus abnormality.

Electrical stimulation of the rectal mucosa in patients and control subjects produces internal anal sphincter relaxation. The stimulus required to produce maximal anal relaxation is significantly increased in patients with severe constipation which suggests an abnormality in the intramural pathway possibly in the myenteric plexus (Kerrigan *et al.*, 1989, Varma and Smith 1986; Dapoigny *et al.*, 1988).

Preston and Lennard-Jones (1985a, 1985b) have therefore suggested that slow transit patients are either a heterogeneous population or that the myenteric plexus disorder is not the primary cause of the condition especially as myenteric plexus degeneration may be a secondary phenomenon induced by prolonged use of laxatives (Smith 1968) which most of these patients will have swallowed in large quantities.

Nerve fibres within the circular smooth muscle layer of the descending colon normally contain vasoactive intestinal peptide (VIP). In chronically constipated patients the concentrations of VIP and peptide histidine- methionine are reduced in the muscularis externa of specimens of colon obtained during colectomy performed primarily for this problem (Koch *et al.*, 1988). Colonic VIP deficiency may be important in the aetiology of chronic constipation in some but not all patients especially as it is known to be deficient in patients with Hirschsprung's disease.

The mechanism by which VIP may contribute to constipation is still uncertain. VIP may be the non-adrenergic non-cholinergic inhibitory neurotransmitter and is thought to produce relaxation of the circular colonic smooth muscle in the normal individual. Loss of this action would delay colonic transit. VIP deficiency may also be expected to lead to loss of the recto-anal inhibitory reflex as the pathway for relaxation may be lost.

Colonic substance P levels are also reduced in chronic severe constipation (Goldin *et al.*, 1989).

Small bowel transit in idiopathic constipation

The relationship and integration between small and large bowel transit is complex. The ability to measure orocaecal transit times has enabled this to be studied in some detail. The subject has been excellently reviewed by Gilmore (1990).

Bond and Levitt (1975) were the first to demonstrate that pulmonary excretion of hydrogen occurred within ten minutes after the introduction of carbohydrate into the caecum. La Brooy *et al.* (1983) refined the technique and devised the lactulose hydrogen breath test which has become the standard test used for the measurement of orocaecal transit. A test meal is given in which 10–30g lactulose is mixed which is followed by serial measurements of breath hydrogen at five minute intervals.

The breath hydrogen concentration profile exhibits a small early peak in 89% of normal individuals which coincides with the emptying of the remnants of the previous meal from the ileum into the colon (Read *et al.*, 1985). Initially this was considered the cause of the increase but it is now thought to be due to buccal fermentation of ingested carbohydrate, as the early peak can be abolished by a bacterial mouthwash and by duodenal intubation (Mastrapaolo and Rees, 1987).

In normal individuals a second peak, after approximately 80 minutes, coincides with rectal filling. Orocaecal transit time is defined as the time from ingestion of the test meal to the first definite and sustained increase in breath hydrogen. This is normally the second peak.

It has been suggested that orocaecal transit time increases with age as Haboubi *et al.* (1988) found prolonged transit times in elderly patients attending a day hospital. They also found that elderly patients with Parkinsons Disease had even more prolonged orocaecal transit times.

Constipation or faecal loading may affect whole gut transit by means other than pure mechanical obstruction as recent studies have shown that rectal distension may reduce small bowel motility and transit (Youle and Read, 1984; Kellow *et al.*, 1987).

Bannister *et al.* (1986) found that many young women with chronic idiopathic constipation in addition to having prolonged whole gut transit have prolonged orocaecal transit times which appears to be due to a small bowel abnormality as they have normal gastric emptying. Their transit delay is not corrected by emptying the colon. Stivland *et al.* (1991), in their scintigraphic study, found that two of their eight constipated patients had slow small bowel transit and another two had delayed gastric emptying. Others have also demonstrated the link between prolonged small bowel transit and delayed colonic transit in constipated patients (Read *et al.*, 1986a; Cann *et al.*, 1983). This suggests the presence of a generalised intestinal motor dysfunction in these patients.

Gross orocaecal transit delays may produce symptoms as in chronic or recurrent pseudo-obstruction when small bowel bacterial overgrowth may also occur (Anuras and Christiansen, 1981). It appears that the resting interdigestive migrating motor complex is particularly important in 'cleansing' the colon and preventing this colonisation (Vantrappen *et al.*, 1977).

Orocaecal transit times in patients with hyperthyroidism are shortened. There is, however, no change in orocaecal transit times in hypothyroidism (Tobin *et al.*, 1989) which suggests that constipation in these patients is due to delayed colonic transit.

Defaecatory difficulty

The main purpose of propulsive colonic motility or transit is to deliver faeces to the rectum for defaecation. Defaecatory difficulties have been demonstrated in younger women with severe slow transit constipation. Many of these patients are unable to expel simulated stools from the rectum (Preston and Lennard-Jones, 1985b; Barnes and Lennard-Jones, 1985;, Read *et al.*, 1986b) despite being able to raise intrarectal pressure to normal levels (Barnes and Lennard-Jones 1985). They also experience difficulty expelling barium or saline (Turnbull *et al.*, 1986).

Preston and Lennard-Jones (1985b), in a study of 28 chronically constipated patients, all of whom had taken laxatives for many years found a number of differences between slow transit and normal transit patients. Their 19 slow transit patients were unable to expel a water filled balloon from the rectum whereas the nine patients with normal transit were able to expel this balloon. The slow transit patients had normal colonic motility though their motility traces tended to be rather flat. In contrast the patients with normal transit constipation were found to have increased colonic activity which Preston and Lennard-Jones suggested may contribute towards the production of small hard stools and pain in these patients.

Turnbull et al (1988) performed rectal evacuation studies on 58 constipated patients and found considerable variation in normal individuals but they did not differ from constipated patients in their anorectal angle and perineal position or the presence of an anterior rectocele. Seventy eight percent of the constipated patients studied took longer to evacuate barium than the control subjects and 57% did not expel it as completely. No differences, however, were found between slow transit and normal transit patients or between constipated patients who did or did not digitally evacuate the rectum.

Kamm *et al.* (1989a) have quantified rectal evacuation during defaecation by inserting 100mls of barium sulphate paste into the rectum and then asking subjects to evacuate the rectum as rapidly and as completely as possible. Normal subjects are able to evacuate completely and quickly. Severely constipated patients exhibit a variety of evacuation disturbances

Normally during defaecation, intrarectal pressure rises and there is a reduction in anal pressure. A pressure gradient is therefore produced which facilitates expulsion of faeces. The rise in intrarectal pressure may be produced by rectal smooth muscle contraction, contraction of the abdominal muscles and/or diaphragm or a combination of both of these.

Rectal activity has usually been assessed by measuring rectal compliance. The technique used to do this is the proctometrogram (Preston *et al.*, 1983b; Varma and Smith 1986a) which involves the instillation of water into a rectal balloon with a constant rate infusion pump whilst the pressure in the rectal balloon is recorded by a transducer and chart recorder. The slope of the pressure *vs.* volume curve is used to calculate rectal compliance (see Fig 17, p. 34.)

Rectal sensation can also be assessed during this procedure by asking patients to indicate to the examiner when the senations of awareness, call to stool and urgency are experienced.

Rectal compliance in patients with severe constipation is increased as large volumes of water have to be instilled into the rectum to produce small increases in rectal pressure (Read *et al.*, 1986b; Bannister *et al.*, 1986; Varma and Smith, 1985). Rectosigmoid motility usually increases after eating (Roe *et al.*, 1986) but this is less marked in patients with intractable constipation.

Madoff *et al.* (1990) have questioned the relevance of these techniques as they argue that rectal compliance is not accurately measured by balloon distension techniques.

Kumar *et al.* (1989) have used prolonged ambulatory studies of anorectal function to demonstrate the presence of periodic activity in the rectum. They have identified abnormalities in the sampling reflex and phasic rectal motor complexes in patients with slow transit constipation who have a significantly lower frequency of sampling responses (mean = 2.4/hr) compared with control patients (7.4/hr) (Waldron *et al.*, 1990). These sampling responses occur in response to rectal filling with faeces or flatus in a group of patients in whom the recto-anal inhibitory reflex has previously been shown to be normal (Waldron *et al.*, 1988; Read *et al.*, 1986b).

There is therefore now clear evidence of diminished transit of stool not only through the colon but also from the colon into the rectum in these patients (Waldron *et al.*, 1990). Patients with intractable constipation have also been shown to have episodic rectal motor complexes similar to control subjects but these complexes are significantly reduced in amplitude (Waldron *et al.*, 1990). Waldron *et al.* (1990) presumed the complexes represented rectal contractile events which in control subjects play a role in transit or defaecation, or both. They suggest that these may be deficient in constipated patients.

Delayed rectal filling and a motor neuropathy affecting the rectum appear therefore to contribute towards defaecatory difficulty.

Obstructed defaecation

Obstructed defaecation is recognised as another contributory factor in idiopathic constipation (Martelli *et al.*, 1978; Preston *et al.*, 1984a; Bartolo *et al.*, 1983; Roe *et al.*, 1986; Hansen *et al.*, 1987).

In normal defaecation the external sphincter and puborectalis muscles both relax to allow the passage of stool. Patients with obstructed defaecation, however, have been shown to exhibit a paradoxical increase in EMG activity in these muscles on attempted defaecation (Preston and Lennard-Jones, 1985b; Read *et al.*, 1986b; Womack *et al.*, 1985; Kuipers *et al.*, 1986;, Turnbull *et al.*, 1986; Roe *et al.*, 1986). This is similar to the external urethral sphincter contraction that occurs in patients with bladder neck dyssynergia (Robinson, 1984).

Kerrigan *et al.* (1989) suggest that failure of external sphincter relaxation during defaecation occurs in 73% of constipated patients compared with 12% of controls

Bartolo *et al.* (1988) used dynamic evacuation proctography in a study of normal transit constipated patients with obstructed defaecation to identify the following causes:

1. puborectalis accentuation (22%);
2. rectal intussussception (52%);
3. anterior rectal wall prolapse (22%);
4. rectocoele (4%).

Perineal descent was seen in patients with rectal intussusception and anterior wall prolapse, but not in those with the other conditions. Isolated anterior rectal mucosal prolapse, which had been proposed as the cause of obstructive symptoms by Parks *et al.* (1966), was not demonstrated.

Failure of the anorectal angle to open on straining has also been shown in these patients (Preston and Lennard-Jones, 1984a; Womack *et al.*, 1986;, Roe *et al.*, 1986; Read *et al.*, 1986b).

The character of the stool also adds to the difficulties as even normal individuals find it more difficult to pass small hard stools (Read *et al.*, 1986b).

Rectal sensation

Abnormal rectal sensation of distension also appears to contribute towards the development of constipation. Most studies have relied upon balloon distension of the rectum for the assessment of sensation. This technique has, however, been challenged as not being accurate enough as there are too many variables which may affect the results (Madoff *et al.*, 1990).

These techniques have, however, been used to demonstrate significant impairment of rectal sensation of distension causing call to stool in patients with severe constipation (Read *et al.*, 1986b; Shouler and Keighley, 1986; Kamm and Lennard-Jones, 1990). Only 38% of constipated patients perceive a desire to defaecate during rectal distension with up to 100mls (Kerrigan *et al.*, 1989).

De Medici *et al.* (1989) using a balloon distension method demonstrated that the degree of rectal sensory impairment was more pronounced in patients with slow transit constipation especially if the transit delay was principally in the rectum. Rectal sensation was found to improve with the treatment of constipation in those patients who responded to treatment but not in the non-responders.

Kamm and Lennard-Jones, (1990) assessed rectal mucosal electro-sensitivity using a bipolar electrode that supplied a constant current. They found the sensory threshold was significantly elevated in constipated patients compared with a normal control group. There was significant correlation between the sensory thresholds for balloon distension and mucosal electrosensitivity.

There is evidence therefore of a rectal sensory neuropathy. This may be a primary cause of constipation or could be secondary to irreversible damage that occurs secondary to the constipation.

The neuropathy may be due to a deficit in the integration of sensory information within the sacral cord. Kerrigan *et al.* (1989) electrically stimulated the dorsogenital nerve whilst recording the evoked reflex activity in the external and urethral sphincters with concentric needle and surface EMA electrodes. 75% of their constipated patients had absence of one or more of the evoked sacral responses compared with 20% of the controls. Varma and Smith, (1988) arrived at a similar conclusion when they demonstrated prolonged pudendo-anal reflex latencies in association with normal sensory thresholds and motor unit potentials in 15 chronically constipated women.

Absence of these evoked responses suggests a localised anatomical or physiological disruption of neural signals transmitted through the sacral cord segments (Kerrigan *et al.*, 1989; Varma and Smith, 1988).

An alternative explanation is that excessive inhibition of sacral cord function may be in operation as Bradley *et al.* (1985) noted that it was possible for subjects to consciously inhibit electrically evoked sacral reflexes.

Urological problems in constipation

Urological problems are well recognised in young female patients with severe constipation (Bannister *et al.*, 1988; Kerrigan *et al.*, 1989).

Urodynamic abnormalities, e.g. increased bladder capacity, acon-tractile bladder and genuine stress incontinence, were present in 56% of patients in one study (Kerrigan *et al.*, 1989). Bannister *et al.*, (1988) found that bladder sensation was impaired and bladder capacity increased in constipated women compared with normal subjects and that similar problems were also present with rectal function but they found no evidence of bladder outflow obstruction even in the patients with obstructed defaecation.

Megarectum

Megarectum has been found to be present in approximately 10% of patients with chronic idiopathic constipation (Verduron *et al.*, 1988).

Verduron *et al.* (1988) extensively investigated 35 patients with a megarectum. Megarectum was defined as a maximal tolerable volume of rectal distension which exceeds 320mls in women or 440mls in men for which no aetiology had been identified. Seven of their patients had congenital megarectum, i.e. Hirschsprung's disease. All their patients were incontinent of faeces. Segmental colonic transit studies demonstrated that left and right colonic transit was normal but they had a marked rectosigmoid delay. The recto-anal inhibitory reflex is absent in these patients.

There was a female predominance among the patients with late onset megarectum half of whom were faecally incontinent. Rectal sensation was grossly impaired but the rectal pressure at the threshold for sensation was found to be similar to that in normal individuals which suggests that the main abnormality is motor rather than sensory with a marked loss of rectal elasticity. The amplitude of the recto-anal inhibitory reflex is reduced in these patients but it can be induced with increasing rectal distension.

Half the late onset megarectum patients had prolonged whole gut transit times. These physiological abnormalities may all contribute towards outlet obstruction leading to megarectum.

Some patients with severe constipation may suffer an intestinal obstruction in the absence of a physical blockage of the colon or small bowel. They may be considered to have an intestinal pseudo-obstruction due to a severe motility abnormality of the gastrointestinal tract. This appears to affect not only the colon but also the upper gastrointestinal tract including the stomach (Mayer *et al.*, 1988; Stanghellini *et al.*, 1987; Reynolds *et al.*, 1987). Reynolds *et al.* (1987) found that 25% of chronically constipated patients had proximal gastrointestinal motility disorders.

Gynaecological problems in constipation

Hormonal and gynaecological abnormalities are recognised in many young women with severe slow transit constipation (Preston and Lennard-Jones, 1986).

Hysterectomy

A number of studies have been performed which have suggested hysterectomy to be a potential cause of constipation (Roe *et al.*, 1988; Taylor *et al.*, 1989; Smith *et al.*, 1990).

Roe *et al.* (1988) studied 31 women with slow transit constipation and found that 14 (45%) had developed severe symptoms after having a hysterectomy. Most of the anorectal physiological measurements were not found to differ between the constipated post hysterectomy patients and the constipated no hysterectomy patients. The authors suggest that parasympathetic nerve fibres may be damaged during hysterectomy which could adversely affect colonic function and cause slow transit constipation.

Taylor *et al.* (1989) studied a series of women who had had a hysterectomy in the previous 24 months and compared them with a matched control group. They found that the hysterectomy patients had a higher incidence of persistent bladder and bowel dysfunction compared with the controls and that the onset of these problems often coincided with the hysterectomy.

Smith *et al.* (1990) followed this study by extensively studying 14 women with profound constipation following hysterectomy and compared them with a group of asymptomatic controls. Twelve of these patients also had severe urinary symptoms e.g. incontinence and retention but the physiological changes were all limited to colon and rectum. Anal physiology was normal. Rectal compliance was increased and rectal sensation was found to be impaired.

In their control group they found that there was a gradient of colonic motility from the proximal to the distal colon which was absent in their constipated patients. Prostigmine stimulation enhanced the gradient in the controls but reversed it in the patients which suggests a functional obstruction in these patients. Smith *et al.* (1990) describe this response as a typical denervation supersensitivity response. The parasympathetic fibres for the bladder and bowel appear therefore to have been damaged at the time of surgery in these patients.

Hormonal effects upon intestinal transit

Studies that have examined the effects of the sex hormones on bowel function and intestinal transit have not revealed any changes during the menstrual cycle in either normal or constipated patients (Kamm *et al.*, 1989b; Turnbull *et al.*, 1989). There is, however, a reduction in the levels of adrenal and to a lesser extent ovarian steroid hormones in severely constipated women (Kamm *et al.*, 1991). The pituitary hormones were normal. These changes were not thought likely to account for the motility disturbance in these constipated patients.

Constipation and haemorrhoids

The relationship between haemorrhoids and constipation has been investigated by Gibbons *et al.* (1988) as it has been suggested that constipation causes haemorrhoids. Prolapsing haemorrhoids, however, were not present in any of their constipated patients but they did find that anal resting pressure was considerably increased in their patients with haemorrhoids compared to both normal subjects and constipated patients. This may be due to the increased vascular pressure within the anal cushions (Sun *et al.*, 1990).

Psychiatric symptoms in constipation

Wald *et al.* (1989) studied 25 severely constipated patients, ten of whom had normal transit and 15 slow transit constipation. They found psychological problems to be greater among the normal transit patients than among the slow transit patients. Wald *et al.* postulated that psychological abnormalities lead patients to seek help. Their bowel habit may be normal but is perceived otherwise by these patients. The treatment for these patients should therefore be based upon behavioural management.

Psychological abnormalities are, however, recognised in many patients with intractable slow transit constipation (Preston *et al.*, 1984b). These may occur secondary to the bowel problems though the alternative explanation, that constipation is a complication of their underlying psychiatric illness or its treatment, is often true.

Drug induced constipation

Constipation may occur secondary to treatment with many drugs among which opiate analgesics are perhaps the most common.

References

Anuras S, Christiansen J. (1981). Recurrent or chronic intestinal pseudo obstruction. *Gastroenterol*; **10**: 177–89.

Bannister JJ, Lawrence WT, Smith A, Thomas DG, Read NW. (1988) Urological abnormalities in young women with severe constipation. *Gut*; **29**: 17–20.

Bannister JJ, Timms JM, Barfield LJ, Donnelly TC, Read NW. (1986) Physiological studies in young women with chronic constipation. *Int J Colorect Dis*; **1**: 175–82.

Barnes PRH, Lennard-Jones JE. (1985) Balloon expulsion from the rectum in constipation of different types. *Gut*; **26**: 1049–1052.

Bartolo DCC, Read NW, Jarratt JA, Read MG, Donnelly TC, Johnson AG. (1983) Differences in anal sphincter function and clinical presentation in patients with pelvic floor descent. *Gastroenterology*; **85**: 68–75.

Bartolo DCC, Roe AM, Virjee J, Mortensen NJMcC, Locke-Edmunds JC. (1988) An analysis of rectal morphology in obstructed defaecation. *Int J Colorect Dis*; **3**: 17–22.

Bassotti G, Gaburri M, Imbimbo BP, *et al.*, (1988) Colonic mass movements in idiopathic chronic constipation. *Gut*; **29**: 1173–9.

Bazzocchi G, Ellis J, Villanueva-Meyer J, *et al.*, (1990). Postprandial colonic transit and motor activity in chronic constipation. *Gastroenterology*; **98**: 686–93.

Bond JH, Levitt MD. (1975) Investigation of small bowel transit time in man utilising pulmonary hydrogen (H_2) measurement. *J Lab Clin Med*; **85**: 546–55.

Bradley WE, Brantley Scott F, Timm GW. (1985) Sphincter electromyelography. *Urol Clin N Am*; **1**: 69–80.

Cann PA, Read NW, Brown C, Hobson N, Holdsworth CD. (1983) Irritable bowel syndrome: relatioship of disorders in the transit of a single meal to symptom patterns. *Gut*; **24**: 405–11.

Chaussade S, Khyari A, Roche H, *et al.*, (1989) Determination of total and segmental colonic transit time in constipated patients. Results in 91 patients with a new simplified method. *Dig Dis Sci*; **34**: 1168–72.

Dapoigny M, Trolese JF, Bommelaer G, Tournot R. (1988) Myoelectric spiking activity of right colon, left colon and rectosigmoid of healthy humans. *Dig Dis Sci*; **33**: 1007–12.

De Medici A, Badiali D, Corazziari E, Bausano G, Anzini F. (1989) Rectal sensitivity in chronic constipation. *Dig Dis Sci*; **34**: 747–753.

Gibbons CP, Bannister JJ, Read NW. (1988) Role of constipation and anal hypertonia in the pathogenesis of haemorrhoids. *Br J Surg*; **75**: 656–60.

Gilmore IT. (1990) Orocaecal transit time in health and disease. *Gut*; **31**: 250–1.

Goldin E, Karmeli F, Selinger Z, Rachmilewitz D. (1989) Colonic substance P levels are increased in ulcerative colitis and decreased in chronic severe constipation. *Dig Dis Sci*; **34**: 754–7.

Haboubi NY, Hudson P, Rahman Q, Lee GS, Ross A. (1988) Small intestinal transit time in the elderly. *Lancet*; **i**: 933.

Hansen FC, Ensor R, Marcum S, Schuster MM. (1987) Diagnostic and physiologic usefulness of the videoproctogram. *Gastroenterology*; **92**: 1425.

Hardcastle JD, Mann CV. (1968) Study of large bowel peristalsis. *Gut*; **9**: 512–20.

Huizinga JD, Daniel EE. (1986) Control of human colonic motor function. *Dig Dis Sci*; **31**: 865–77.

Kamm MA, Bartram CI, Lennard-Jones JE. (1989a) Rectodynamics – quantifying rectal evacuation. *Int J Colorect Dis*; **4**: 161–3.

Kamm MA, Farthing MJG, Lennard-Jones JE. (1989b) Bowel function and transit rate during the menstrual cycle. *Gut*; **30**: 605–8.

Kamm MA, Farthing MJG, Lennard-Jones JE, Perry LA, Chard T. (1991) Steroid hormone abnormalities in women with severe idiopathic constipation. *Gut*; **34**: 80–4.

Kamm MA, Lennard-Jones JE. (1990) Rectal mucosal electrosensory testing – evidence of a rectal sensory neuropathy in idiopathic constipation. *Dis Colon Rectum*; **33**: 429–33.

Kamm MA, Lennard-Jones JE, Thompson DG, Sobnack R, Garvie NW, Gransowska M. (1988) Dynamic scanning defines a colonic defect in severe idiopathic constipation. *Gut*; **29**: 1085–92.

Kellow JE, Gill RC, Wingate DL. (1987) Modulation of human upper gastrointestinal motility by rectal distension. *Gut*; **28**: 864–8.

Kerrigan DD, Lucas MG, Sun WM, Donelly TC, Read NW. (1989) Idiopathic constipation associated with impaired urethrovesical and sacral reflex function. *Br J Surg*; **76**: 748–51.

Koch TR, Carney A, GO L, Go VLW. (1988) Idiopathic chronic constipation is associated with decreased colonic vasoactive intestinal peptide. *Gastroenterology*; **94**: 300–10.

Krishnamurphy S, Schniffer MD, Rohrmann CA, Ope CE. (1985) Severe idiopathic constipation is associated with a distinctive abnormality of the colonic myenteric plexus. *Gastroenterology*; **88**: 26–34.

Kuipers HC, Bleijeuberg G, Morree HDE. (1986) The spastic pelvic floor syndrome. Large bowel outlet obstruction caused by pelvic floor dysfunction: A radiological study. *Int J Colorect Dis*; **1**: 44–8.

Kumar D, Williams NS, Waldron DJ, Wingate DL. (1989) Prolonged manometric recording of anorectal motor activity in ambulant human subjects: evidence of periodic motor activity. *Gut*; **30**: 1007–11.

La Brooy SJ, Male PJ, Beavis AK, Misiewicz JJ. (1983) Assessment of the reproducibility of the lactulose H2 breath test as a measure of mouth to caecum transit time. *Gut*. **24**: 893–6.

Lanfranchi GA, Bazzocchi G, Brignola C, Campieri M, Labo G. (1984) Different patterns of intestinal transit time and anorectal motility in painful and painless chronic constipation. *Gut*; **25**: 1352–7.

Madoff RD, Orrom WJ, Rothenberger DA, Goldberg SM. (1990) Rectal compliance: a critical reappraisal. *Int J Colorect Dis*; **5**: 37–40.

Martelli H, Devroede G, Arhan P, Duguay C, Dornic C, Faverdin C. (1978). Mechanism of idiopathic constipation: outlet obstruction. *Gastroenterology*; **75**: 623–31.

Mastrapaolo G, Rees WDW. (1987) Evaluation of the hydrogen breath test in man: definition and elimination of the early hydrogen peak. *Gut*; **28**: 721–5.

Mayer EA, Elashoff J, Hawkins R, Berquist W, Taylor IL. (1988) Gastric emptying of mixed solid-liquid meal in patients with intestinal pseudoobstruction. *Dig Dis Sci*; **33**: 10–18.

Metcalf AM, Phillips SF, Zinsmeister Ar, MacCarty RL, Beart RW, Wolff BG. (1987) Simplified assessment of segmental colonic transit. *Gastroenterology*; **92**: 40–7.

Meunier P, Rochas A, Lambert R. (1979) Motor activity of the sigmoid colon in chronic constipation: comparative study with normal subjects. *Gut*; **20**: 1095–1101.

Parks AG, Porter NH, Hardcastle J. (1966) The syndrome of the descending perineum. *Proc Roy Soc Med*; **59**: 477–82.

Preston DM. (1985) Arbuthnot Lane's disease; chronic intestinal stasis. *Br J Surg*; **72(Suppl)**: S8–S10.

Preston DM, Barnes PRH, Lennard-Jones JE. (1983a) Proctometrogram: does it have a role in the evaluation of adults with constipation? **Gut**; **24**: A1010–A1011.

Preston DM, Butler MG, Smith B, Lennard-Jones JE. (1983b) Neuropathology of slow transit constipation. *Gut*; **24**: A997.

Preston DM, Lennard-Jones JE. (1985a) Pelvic colon motility and response to intraluminal bisacodyl in slow transit constipation. *Dig Dis Sci*; **30**: 289–94.

Preston DM, Lennard-Jones JE. (1985b) Anismus in chronic constipation. *Dig Dis Sci*; **30**: 413–18.

Preston DM, Lennard-Jones JE. (1986) Severe chronic constipation of young women: 'idiopathic slow transit constipation'. *Gut*; **27**: 41–8.

Preston DM, Lennard-Jones JE, Thomas BM. (1984a) The balloon proctogram. *Br J Surg*; **71**: 29–32.

Preston DM, Pfeffer JM, Lennard-Jones JE. (1984b). Psychiatric assessment of patients with severe constipation. *Gut*; **25**: A582–3.

Read NW, Al-Janabi MN, Bates TE, *et al.* (1985) Interpretation of the breath hydrogen profile obtained after ingesting a solid meal containing unabsorbable carbohydrate. *Gut*; **26**: 834–42.

Read NW, Al-Janabi MN, Holgate AM, Barber DC, Edwards CA. (1986a) Simultaneous measurement of gastric emptying, small bowel residence and colonic filling of a solid meal by the use of the gamma camera. *Gut*; **27**: 300–8.

Read NW, Timms JM, Barfield LJ, Donnelly TC, Bannister JJ. (1986b). Impairment of defaecation in young women with severe constipation. *Gastroenterology*; **90**: 53–60.

Reynolds JC, Ouyang A, Lee CA, Baker L, Sunshine AG, Cohen S. (1987) Chronic severe constipation. Prospective studies in 25 consecutive patients. *Gastroenterology*; **92**: 414–20.

Robinson JM. (1984) Evaluation of methods for assessment of bladder and urethral function. In: Brocklehurst JC (ed) *Urology in the Elderly*; pp 19–54. Churchill Livingstone, Edinburgh.

Roe AM, Bartolo DCC, Mortensen NJMcC. (1986) Diagnosis and surgical management of intractable constipation. *Br J Surg*; **73**: 854–61.

Roe AM, Bartolo DCC, McC Mortensen NJ. (1988) Slow transit constipation. Comparison between patients with or without previous hysterectomy. *Dig Dis Sci*; **33** 1159–63.

Shouler P, Keighley MRB. (1986) Changes in colonic function in severe idiopathic chronic constipation. *Gastroenterology*; **90**: 414–20.

Smith B. (1968) Effect of irritant purgatives on the myenteric plexus in man and the mouse. *Gut*; **9**: 139–143.

Smith AN, Varma JS, Binnie NR, Papachrysostomou M. (1990) Disordered colorectal motility in intractable constipation following hysterectomy. *Br J Surg*; **77**: 1361–66.

Stanghellini V, Camilleri M, Malagelada JR. (1987) Chronic idiopathic intestinal psuedo-obstruction: clinical and intestinal manometric findings. *Gut;* **28:** 5–12.

Stivland T, Camilleri M, Vassallo M, Proano M, Rath D, Brown M, Thomforde G, Pemberton J, Phillips SF. (1991) Scintigraphic measurement of regional gut transit inidiopathic constipation. *Gastroenterology;* **101:** 107–115.

Sun WM, Read NW, Shorthouse AJ. (1990) Hypertensive anal cushions as a cause of the high anal canal pressures in patients with haemorrhoids. *Br J Surg;* **77:** 458–462.

Taylor T, Smith AN, Fulton PM. (1989) Effect of hysterectomy on bowel function. *Br Med J;* **299:** 300–1.

Tobin MV, Fisken RA, Diggory RT, Morris AI, Gilmore IT. (1989) Orocaecal transit time in health and in thyroid disease. *Gut;* **30:** 26–9.

Turnbull GK, Bartram CI, Lennard-Jones JE. (1988) Radiologic studies of rectal evacuation in adults with idiopathic constipation. *Dis Colon Rectum;* **31:** 190–7.

Turnbull GK, Lennard-Jones JE, Bartram CI. (1986) Failure of rectal expulsion as a cause of constipation: why fibre and laxatives sometimes fail. *Lancet;* **i:** 767–9.

Turnbull GK, Thompson DG, Day S, Martin J, Walker E, Lennard-Jones JE. (1989) Relationships between symptoms, menstrual cycle and orocaecal transit in normal and constipated women. *Gut;* **30:** 30–4.

Vantrappen G, Janssens J, Ghoos Y. (1977) The interdigestive motor complex of normal subjects and patients with bacterial overgrowth of the small intestine. *J Cli Invest;* **59:** 1158–66.

Varma JS, Smith AN. (1986) Reproducibility of the proctometrogram. *Gut;* **27:** 288–92.

Varma JS, Smith AN. (1986) Anorectal function following anal sleeve anastomosis for chronic radiation injury to the rectum. *Br J Surg;* **73:** 285–9.

Varma JS, Smith AN. (1988) Neurophysiological dysfunction in young women with intractable constipation. *Gut;* **29:** 963–8.

Varma JS, Smith AN, Smith RG, Bradnock J. (1985) Colorectal function in the elderly constipated. *Gut;* **26:** A573.

Verduron A, Devroede G, Bouchoucha M, *et al.* (1988) Megarectum. *Dig Dis Sci;* **33:** 1164–74.

Wald A, Hinds JP, Caruana BJ. (1989) Psychological and physiological characteristics of patients with severe idiopathic constipation. *Gastroenterology;* **97:** 932–7.

Waldron DJ, Bowes KL, Kingma YT, Cote K. (1988) Colonic and anorectal motility in young women with severe constipation. *Gastroenterology;* **95:** 1388–94.

Waldron DJ, Kumar D, Hallan RI, Wingate DL, Williams NS. (1990) Evidence for motor neuropathy and reduced filling of the rectum in chronic intractable constipation. *Gut;* **31:** 1284–8.

Womack NR, Morrison JFB, Williams NS. (1986) The role of pelvic floor denervation in the aetiology of idiopathic faecal incontinence. *Br J Surg;* **73:** 404–7.

Womack NR, Williams NS, Holmfield JHM, Morrison JFB, Simpkins KC. (1985) New method for the dynamic assessment of anorectal function in constipation. *Br J Surg;* **72:** 994–8.

Youle MS, Read NW. (1984) Effect of painless rectal distension on gastrointestinal transit of solid meal. *Dig Dis Sci;* **29:** 902–6.

12

Constipation in the elderly

Constipation in the elderly may be the presenting symptom of colonic disease. The possible causes are listed in Table 1, p. 87. These include drugs especially those with constipating effects, e.g. morphine and other opiate analgesics. Laxative use may also contribute towards constipation in some patients by producing dehydration, hypokalaemia or myenteric plexus degeneration (Smith, 1968).

Constipation is common in immobile elderly patients (Donald et al., 1985) probably because their ability to respond to the call to stool is impaired as a result of their poor mobility and their need for assistance with toileting. Resende (1989), in a study of 400 elderly immobile patients in hospital continuing care beds, found that the frequency of defaecation was related to patients' mobility, activities of daily living score, mental status score, hearing and speech problems. Other physiological causes may be present in these patients. This will be discussed later in this chapter.

Constipation in the elderly does not appear to differ in prevalence between the sexes unlike the situation in younger patients in whom there is a strong female bias. The larger number of elderly females with the problem purely reflect the overall population sex difference in old age.

Diagnosis

The methods used to diagnose constipation in the elderly were evaluated in a community survey by Donald et.al. (1985). Using abdominal radiography as the final arbiter, they considered true constipation was present in less than half of their patients complaining of constipation. Straining at stool was the only symptom that they found to be associated with radiographic evidence of colonic faecal loading. They also confirmed that the presence of some faeces in the rectum is not necessarily abnormal.

Donald *et.al.* suggested that digital rectal examination was unreliable as a true indicator of constipation as the amount of faeces on rectal examination did not correlate with either colonic loading on the radiograph or the symptoms of constipation. They did not, however, correlate it with rectal faecal loading for which it is still the quickest method of diagnosis and also the most relevant when considering the management of constipation and faecal impaction.

In clinical practice an abdominal radiograph is not always required in the assessment of the constipation but may be useful in the detection of high faecal loading, i.e. colonic, in the absence of rectal loading (Smith and Lewis, 1990).

Pain does not appear to be a major factor of constipation in the elderly but no formal prevalence study has been performed.

Definition

Constipation is a term normally used to indicate either the infrequent passage of stool (two or fewer stools passed per week) or excessive straining on attempted defaecation.

Faecal impaction is the main feature of constipation in the elderly and is frequently associated with faecal incontinence. Read *et.al.* (1985) found that 42% of the admissions to an acute geriatric ward were impacted with faeces which they defined as the presence of hard masses of faeces within the rectum. Some old people with faecal impaction may, however, present atypically as they may continue to have a bowel action(s) every day or present with incontinence of urine, faeces or both. Spurious diarrhoea may also occur. This term, however, is misleading for many clinicians consider it to refer to loose stool passing around a hard mass of faeces in the rectum. This occurs much less frequently than the rectum being loaded with a large amount of soft or liquid faeces.

Most physicians use the term faecal impaction to describe faecal loading of the rectum and/or colon with hard stool usually in patients with a history of chronic constipation. Many elderly patients, however, would be excluded by this definition as they develop massive faecal loading with soft or liquid stool (Barrett, 1988a).

Barrett (1988b) reported that 45% of the faecally loaded patients in his study had large amounts of soft or liquid stool in the rectum. The remaining patients were loaded with stool which was firm in consistency. Only 10% of the overall total had rock hard pellets of faeces (scybala) present. Faecal impaction may therefore be better defined as faecal loading of the rectum and/or colon with a large amount of stool of any consistency. Frequently this occurs as a result of an immobilising illness, e.g. stroke, in the absence of a history of chronic constipation.

An important question that remains to be answered is 'why is the faeces of constipated elderly people soft?' Laxatives especially osmotic laxatives and excess fibre intake may be responsible. Once they have been excluded the possible causes may include excess faecal bile acid especially as Nagengast *et.al.* (1988) demonstrated that faecal bile acid concentration increases with age. High concentration of these acids would be expected to lead to loose stools. They suggest that this is due to reduced fibre intake with increasing age but this subject needs further investigation.

Other causes such as fat malabsorption, bacterial overgrowth and other causes of chronic diarrhoea have not been investigated.

Pathophysiology of constipation

The main body of pathophysiological information on idiopathic constipation is derived from studies performed on constipated young women. A few studies of elderly constipated patients have now been performed to supplement these.

Colonic propulsion

The importance of physical activity and eating for normal bowel habit has already been discussed in Chapter 5. It is not surprising therefore that people with severe mobility problems, irrespective of their age, tend to have severe problems with constipation.

Immobility has been shown to be the most important contributory factor in the development of both constipation (Donald *et al.*, 1985) and faecal incontinence in the elderly (Barrett *et.al.* 1988; Barrett 1988b). It has been suggested that the mechanism is likely to be a reduction in the colonic mass movements that Holdstock *et.al.* (1970) have demonstrated are normally induced by physical activity, but no specific studies have been performed to confirm this. A significant reduction in these movements has, however, been demonstrated in young constipated patients (Bassotti *et al.*, 1987).

Poor appetite and food intake may also reduce colonic propulsive motility. Evidence from studies performed on younger patients suggests that the usual postprandial increase in rectosigmoid motility is less marked in constipated patients than in normal individuals (Roe *et.al.*, 1986).

Whole gut transit time is often used to assess the effectiveness of colonic propulsion and defaecation. It does not appear to change with age (see Chapter 7).

Intestinal transit studies have also been performed on the elderly. Brocklehurst and Khan (1969) compared eight immobile elderly patients from long stay geriatric wards with four non-hospitalised active elderly people. They found that all of the control subjects had passed all of the markers by the seventh day which may therefore be regarded as normal. Only one of the long stay patients, however, had passed 80% of the markers by the seventh day though all had passed 80% by the fourtheenth day. In a further study, 37 long stay geriatric patients were all found to have 80% transit times in excess of six days and 30% of them still had markers in situ after 14 days (Brocklehurst *et.al.*, 1983). In the majority of cases the markers reach the descending colon fairly rapidly but are then held up in the rectum and sigmoid colon ((Brocklehurst *et.al.*, 1983; Eastwood 1972). They may thus be described as suffering from the 'terminal reservoir syndrome' a term first used by Bodian *et.al.* (1949).

A myenteric plexus abnormality has been proposed as a contributory factor in slow transit constipation (see p. 89). Primary myenteric plexus degeneration may be the cause of the constipation (Preston and Lennard-Jones, 1985a) or the changes may be secondary to prolonged use of laxatives (Smith, 1968; Preston *et al.*, 1983). Secondary myenteric plexus degeneration has also been described after section of the pelvic nerves (Devroede and Lamarche, 1974) and in patients with spinal cord injuries (Devroede *et.al.*, 1979). There are, however, no studies of myenteric plexus morphology in constipation in the elderly and/or disabled.

The sigmoid colon and rectum therefore appear to be the main sites of delayed gut transit in constipated geriatric patients (Brocklehurst *et al.*, 1983). This may be due to mechanical obstruction by impacted faecal masses in the rectum but other mechanisms may be in operation.

Small bowel motility and transit abnormalities in young constipated women were discussed in Chapter 11. Similar studies of small bowel function have not yet been performed in elderly constipated patients. Delayed colonic and small bowel transit may be secondary to a generalised abnormality within the enteric nervous system, of which the myenteric plexus is of course an integral part.

Defaecatory difficulty

Defaecatory difficulty is well documented in young women with severe slow transit constipation and is demonstrated by their inability to expel simulated stools from the rectum (Preston and Lennard-Jones, 1985b; Barnes and Lennard-Jones, 1985; Read *et.al.*, 1986a).

The ability to defaecate is related to the character of the stool as even normal individuals may find it difficult to expel small hard stools (Bannister *et.al.*, 1987b). Simulated defaecation studies performed on healthy elderly subjects have revealed that although they are able to expel a simulated soft stool (50ml balloon) voluntarily (Read *et.al.*, 1985) they require longer to achieve this than younger subjects (Bannister *et.al.*, 1987a).

Read *et.al.* (1985) and Read and Abouzekry (1986) also investigated the anorectal function of a selected group of 55 elderly patients with faecal impaction from a geriatric medical unit. All their patients were impacted with hard stool and had experienced defaecatory difficulty for at least five years. Eighty-four percent of their patients were ambulant and mental state was normal in 87%. Only patients who were considered of sufficient mental and physical health to comply with the tests were included in the study. They were compared with 36 age and sex matched controls.

The eldery patients with faecal impaction in the above studies are not fully representative of the whole spectrum of constipated patients one would expect to find in a typical department of geriatric medicine as most of these patients have mobility problems and multiple medical illnesses and many are also mentally confused. The results of this well-conducted study do, however, provide an important insight into abnormalities in defaecation and rectal motility in these patients.

The impacted patients were nearly all able to expel the simulated soft stool (balloon containing 50mls of water) but experienced difficulty expelling the simulated hard stool (small solid 18mm diameter sphere). Only 32% of their patients successfully expelled the simulated hard stool compared with 63% of the control group. This difference, however, did not reach significance (Read *et.al.*, 1985).

Many disabled elderly patients, however, experience difficulty even when stool is soft (personal observations). The most severe defaecatory problems appear to be experienced by severely confused patients but these patients were not included in Read *et.al.*'s (1985) study.

During normal defaecation, intrarectal pressure increases with a reduction in anal pressure to produce a pressure gradient which facilitates expulsion of faeces. The increased intrarectal pressure may be produced by rectal smooth muscle contraction, contraction of the abdominal muscles and diaphragm, or a combination of both.

The contribution of increases in intrarectal pressure towards defaecation in the elderly has not been specifically studied. Rectal motility, however, appears to be reduced in old age. Read *et.al.* (1985) were able to elicit regular rectal contractions in response to rectal distension in only 10% of their group of normal elderly people compared with 71% of a group of young healthy subjects who underwent a similar examination in another study (Read *et.al.*, 1986).

Barrett *et.al.* (1990) performed rectal motility studies on disabled elderly patients typical of those managed within a Department of Geriatric Medicine and found that only 13% of the elderly control subjects exhibited rectal contractions during rectal distension which confirmed the results obtained by Read *et.al.* (1985).

Barrett *et.al.* (1990) found that the incidence of multiple or regular rectal contractions following rectal distension did not differ between faecally impacted patients (25%) and the controls (13%). These findings are again similar to those of Read *et.al.* (1985), i.e. 14% and 10% respectively. Thirty-six percent of Read *et.al.*'s (1986) younger constipated patients exhibited these contractions.

Some patients exhibit just a single rectal contraction that occurs at the time of the initial rectal distension. Barrett *et.al.* (1990) found that rectal distension failed to elicit any rectal contractions in 44% of elderly faecally impacted patients and in 58% of their control patients.

Read *et.al.* (1985) were also unable to elicit contractions in 36% of their elderly impacted patients and in 25% of their control subjects. They also found that higher distending volumes were required to elicit rectal contractions in elderly impacted patients than in the controls, though similar studies performed on younger constipated patients produced normal results (Roe *et.al.*, 1986; Read *et.al.*, 1986).

Read *et.al.* (1985) also found that the steady state rectal pressure recorded during rectal distension with a balloon containing 150mls of air was significantly lower in impacted patients than in the controls and that a higher volume of distension is required to produce a steady state pressure of 25 cmH$_2$O. This suggests an increase in rectal compliance in these patients. Similar studies on younger patients with severe constipation have not shown any difference from normal subjects (Roe *et.al.*, 1986; Read *et al.*, 1986).

Varma *et al.* (1988) have suggested that rectal compliance is increased in constipated patients which is supported by Read *et.al.*'s (1985) results.

Barrett *et.al.* (1990), however performed proctometrograms to measure rectal compliance in impacted patients and controls and found no difference between the two groups, which is similar to the result obtained by Bannister *et.al.*, (1986) in a study of young women with chronic constipation. It seems unlikely therefore that rectal compliance is abnormal in impacted geriatric patients, especially as Varma *et.al.* (1988) were also unable to detect any difference in rectal compliance in the group of constipated old people that they compared with an elderly control group.

Varma *et.al.* (1988) suggested, however, that there may be two distinct groups of elderly constipated patients: one group of patients with high compliance (megarectum presumably associated with a myenteric plexus abnormality); and another group with a hypertonic rectal motility response. Although the division of patients into these two groups is rather arbitrary it suggests that there is a heterogeneous mixture of motility disorders contributing towards the development of constipation and faecal impaction in the elderly.

If rectal motility is deficient one might expect a greater contribution from voluntary increases in intra-abdominal pressure to increase intra- rectal pressure for defaecation to proceed. Young constipated patients retain the ability to increase intrarectal pressure voluntarily (Barnes and Lennard-Jones, 1985). No data is available about this in the elderly but one might anticipate this to be impaired. In some elderly patients weakness of the abdominal musculature due to either age related changes in the muscles (probably secondary to denervation) or disuse (particularly in immobile patients) could limit this ability but this has not been studied.

Obstructed defaecation

Normally during defaecation the internal and external anal sphincters and puborectalis muscles relax to allow the passage of stool. The paradoxical increase in the activity of these muscles during attempted defaecation which obstructs defaecation in many young constipated patients (Roe *et.al.*, 1986; Preston and Lennard Jones, 1985b; Read *et.al.*, 1986; Turnbull *et.al.*, 1986; Womack *et.al.*, 1985: Kuipers *et.al.*, 1986) has been discussed in Chapter 11. Detailed defaecatory studies have not been performed on elderly constipated patients.

It has also been suggested that failure of the internal sphincter to relax, as in Hirshsprung's disease (Lawson and Nixon, 1967) could cause defaecatory difficulty. A normal recto-anal inhibitory reflex in response to rectal distension has, however, been demonstrated in both elderly impacted patients (Read and Abouzekry 1986) and in young chronically constipated patients (Bannister *et.al.*, 1986; Read and Abouzekry, 1986).

Failure of the anorectal angle to open on defaecatory straining has also been demonstrated in these young patients (Roe *et al.*, 1986; Read *et al.*, 1986; Preston *et al.*, 1984; Womack *et al.*, 1986). In elderly impacted patients, however, although the angle is obtuse at rest, it appears to increase on straining (Read and Abouzekry, 1986).

Megacolon and pseudo-obstruction

Acquired megacolon and intestinal pseudo-obstruction have been discussed in Chapter 11. Idiopathic intestinal pseudo-obstruction as an acute syndrome has been described mainly in the old and chronically ill, often associated with the development of a megacolon (Bardsley, 1974). Usually there are signs of intestinal obstruction without evidence of a lesion obstructing the intestinal lumen (Faulk *et.al.*, 1978). Gurll and Steer (1975) described a series of patients in whom the clinical presentation was indistinguishable from that of intestinal obstruction due to other causes. A plain abdominal radiograph was the most helpful diagnostic feature, showing faeces throughout the whole colon.

References

Bannister JJ, Davison P, Timms JM, Gibbons C, Read NW. (1987a) Effect of stool size and consistency on defaecation. *Gut*; **28**: 1246–50.

Bannister JJ, Gibbons C, Read NW. (1987b) Preservation of faecal continence during rises in intra-abdominal pressure; is there a role for the flap valve? *Gut*; **28**: 1242–5.

Bannister JJ, Timms JM, Barfield LJ, Donnelly TC, Read NW. (1986) Physiological studies in young women with chronic constipation. *Int J Colorect Dis*; **1**: 175–82.

Bardsley D. (1974) Pseudo-obstruction of the large bowel. *Br J Surg*; **61**: 963–9.

Barnes PRH, Lennard-Jones JE. (1985) Balloon expulsion from the rectum in constipation of different types. *Gut*; **26**: 1049–52.

Barrett JA. (1988a) Effect of wheat bran on weight of stool. *Br Med J*; **296**: 1127–8.

Barrett JA. (1988b) A study of the anorectal pathophysiology of geriatric patients with faecal incontinence. MD thesis. University of Liverpool.

Barrett JA, Brocklehurst JC, Kiff ES, Ferguson G, Faragher EB. (1990) Rectal motility studies in geriatric patients with faecal incontinence. *Age and Ageing*; **19**: 311–17.

Barrett JA, Faragher EB, Kiff ES, Ferguson G, Brocklehurst JC. (1988c) Why are geriatric patients incontinent of faeces? *Clin Sci*; **75**(Suppl 19): 10 p.

Bassotti G, Gaburri M, Imbimbo B, Pelli MA, Morelli A. (1987) Colonic mass movements in health and in constipation. *Gastroenterology*; **92**: 1310.

Bodian M, Stephens FD, Ward BCH. (1949) Hirschsprungs disease and idio-pathic megacolon. *Lancet*; **i**: 6–11

Brocklehurst JC, Khan MY. (1969) A study of faecal stasis in old age and the use of 'Dorbanex' in its prevention. *Gerontol Clin*; **11**: 293–300.

Brocklehurst JC, Kirkland JL, Martin J, Ashford J. (1983) Constipation in long-stay elderly patients: its treatment and prevention by lactulose, poloxalkol-dihydroxyanthroquinolone and phosphate enemas. *Gerontology*; **29**: 181–4.

Devroede G, Arhan P, Duguay C, Tetreault L, Akanry M, Percy B. (1979) Traumatic constipation. *Gastroenterology*; **77**: 1258–67.

Devroede G, Lamarche J. (1974) Functional importance of extrinsic parasympathetic innervation of the distal colon and rectum in man. *Gastroenterology*; **66**: 273–80.

Donald IP, Smith RG, Cruikshank JG, Elton RA, Stoddart ME. (1985) A study of constipation in the elderly living at home. *Gerontology*; **31**: 112–8.

Eastwood HDH. (1972) Bowel transit studies in the elderly: radioopaque markers in the investigation of constipation. *Gerontol Clin*; **14**: 154–9.

Faulk DL, Anuras S, Christensen J. (1978) Chronic intestinal pseudo- obstruction. *Gastroenterology*; **74**: 922–31.

Gurll N, Steer M. (1975) Diagnostic and therapeutic considerations for faecal impaction. *Dis Colon Rectum*; **18**: 507–11.

Holdstock DJ, Misiewicz JJ, Smith T, Rowlands EN. (1970) Propulsion (mass movements) in the human colon and its relationship to meals and somatic activity. *Gut*; **11**: 91–9.

Kuipers HC, Bleijeuberg G, Morree HDE. (1986) The spastic pelvic floor syndrome. Large bowel outlet obstruction caused by pelvic floor dysfunction: A radiological study. *Int J Colorect Dis*; **1**: 44–8.

Lawson JN, Nixon HH. (1967) Anal canal pressures in the diagnosis of Hirschsprung's disease. *J Paediat Surg*; **2**: 544–52.

Nagengast FM, Van Der Werf SDJ, Lamers HLM, Hectors MPC, Buys WCAM, Van Tonergen JMH. (1988) Influence of age, intestinal transit time, and dietary composition on faecal bile acid profiles in healthy subjects. *Dig Dis Sci*; **33**: 673–8.

Preston DM, Butler MG, Smith B, Lennard-Jones JE. (1983) Neuropathology of slow transit constipation. *Gut*; **24**: A997.

Preston DM, Lennard-Jones JE, Thomas BM (1984a) The balloon proctogram. *Br J Surg*; **71**: 29–32.

Preston DM, Lennard-Jones JE. (1985a) Pelvic colon motility and response to intraluminal bisacodyl in slow transit constipation. *Dig Dis Sci*; **30**: 289–94.

Preston DM, Lennard-Jones JE. (1985b) Anismus in chronic constipation. *Dig Dis Sci*; **30**: 413–18.

Read NW, Abouzekry L. (1986) Why do patients with faecal impaction have faecal incontinence. *Gut*; **27**: 283–7.

Read NW, Abouzekry L, Read MG, Howell P, Ottewell D, Donnelly TC. (1985) Anorectal function in elderly patients with faecal impaction. *Gastroenterology*; **89**: 959–66.

Read NW, Timms JM, Barfield LJ, Donnelly TC, Bannister JJ. (1986) Impairment of defaecation in young women with severe constipation. *Gastroenterology*; **90**: 53–60.

Resende TL. (1989) Constipation, faecal incontinence and the effects of exercise and abdominal massage on colonic activity in old age. MSc Thesis, University of Manchester.

Roe AM, Bartolo DCC, Mortensen NJMcC. (1986) Diagnosis and surgical management of intractable constipation. *Br J Surg*; **73**: 854–61.

Smith B. (1968) Effect of irritant purgatives on the myenteric plexus in man and the mouse. *Gut*; **9**: 139–43.

Smith RG, Lewis S. (1990) The relationship between digital rectal examination and abdominal radiographs in elderly patients. *Age and Ageing*; **19**: 142–3.

Turnbull GK, Lennard-Jones JE, Bartram CI. (1986).Failure of rectal expulsion as a cause of constipation: why fibre and laxatives sometimes fail. *Lancet*; **i**: 767–9.

Womack NR, Morrison JFB, Williams NS. (1986) The role of pelvic floor denervation in the aetiology of idiopathic faecal incontinence. *Br J Surg*; **73**: 404–7.

Womack NR, Williams NS, Holmfield JHM, Morrison JFB, Simpkins KC. (1985) New method for the dynamic assessment of anorectal function in constipation. *Br J Surg;* **72**: 994–8.

13

Faecal incontinence secondary to constipation

Constipation is the main cause of faecal incontinence in the elderly (Brocklehurst, 1985; Barrett *et al.*, 1988; Tobin and Brocklehurst, 1986). Sixty-nine percent of the elderly faecally incontinent patients in one study were found to be faecally loaded (Barrett *et al.*, 1989) though in most of these patients there were co-existent anorectal abnormalities.

Anal manometry

The anal resting and squeeze pressures of continent elderly patients with faecal impaction are similar to those of elderly control subjects (Read *et al.*, 1985, Barrett *et al.*, 1989) and are not altered by disimpaction (Read and Abouzekry 1986).

Faecally incontinent and impacted patients, however, have lower anal resting pressures than continent impacted patients (median 54cm H_2O vs. 78cm H_2O). The incontinent patients have also been found to have significantly lower squeeze pressures (median 22cm H_2O vs. 34cm H_2O) though this may be due to the higher incidence of mental impairment in the incontinent impacted group (Barrett *et al.*, 1988).

There are abnormalities in the recto-anal reflex in faecally impacted patients which may increase the risk of incontinence. The inflation reflex, i.e. reflex contraction of the external sphincter in response to rectal distension is present in only 50% of elderly faecally impacted patients (Read and Abouzekry 1986; Barrett *et al.*, 1989). The inhibitory reflex can be elicited in 89% of continent elderly faecally impacted patients but is present in only 53% of the elderly faecally incontinent patients (Barrett *et al.*, 1989).

Stool consistency

Incontinence may occur when the rectum is loaded with either hard or soft faeces but is more likely to occur when faeces is soft than when it is hard. Rectal distension studies using two different simulated stool models have helped to confirm the clinical observations.

The soft stool model was a condom filled with water via a pump. The condom was easily distensible and had a high compliance value. The firm stool model was a party balloon which was more difficult to distend with air than the condom device and had a low compliance value.

During the respective studies patients were asked to retain the devices within the rectum until they experienced urgency but both devices were frequently expelled before the end of the test. This usually occurred before the sensation of 'call to stool' was experienced. The party balloon was involuntarily expelled less frequently by the incontinent patients (18%) than the condom (67%) which suggests that faecal incontinence is more likely when the consistency of stool in the rectum is liquid than when it is firm. The frequency of involuntary expulsion of the condom in the elderly incontinent patients (67%) was similar to that in the continent impacted patients (65%) (Barrett *et al.*, 1990).

Involuntary expulsion of the firm stool model, i.e. party balloon, occurred rarely in the continent impacted patients (4%) which suggests that although these patients are continent of formed stool they would be at risk of incontinence if they developed diarrhoea or were treated with stool softeners or laxatives.

Anorectal angle

The anorectal angle has been found to be more obtuse in elderly patients with faecal impaction than in elderly control subjects (Read and Abouzekry, 1986). One might therefore expect this to be associated with faecal incontinence as the angle is important in the maintenance of continence.

Rectal sensation

There is reasonable evidence of impaired rectal sensation in elderly faecally impacted patients. Two studies have demonstrated that significantly higher volumes of rectal distension are required to produce the desire to defaecate in these patients than in elderly controls (Read and Abouzekry, 1986; Read *et al.*, 1985; Varma *et al.*, 1988). Barrett *et al.* (1990) found similar results in faecally impacted patients but the difference did not quite reach significance (p = 0.06) probably due to the relatively small sample number of faecally impacted patients studied (n = 16).

Many faecally incontinent patients irrespective of their age, are unaware of faecal leakage until after the event, despite 'normal' rectal sensation (Rogers *et al.*, 1988; Barrett *et al.*, 1990; Ferguson *et al.*, 1989). Five of the 30 elderly faecally incontinent patients who had proctometrograms performed by Barrett *et al.* (1990) involuntarily expelled the rectal balloon before the onset of rectal sensation.

The contribution made by rectal sensation to the maintenance of continence may be more complex than just being able to sense rectal distension. Buser and Miner's (1986) observation that rectal sensation is delayed in younger incontinent patients and that relaxation of the anal sphincter occurs before the onset of rectal sensation suggests that the anal sphincter response to rectal distension before the onset of rectal sensation determines whether continence is maintained.

Absence of the inflation reflex (external sphincter contraction) in approximately 50% of the elderly (Barrett *et al.*, 1990) (see p. 65) deprives them of the usual reflex protection that occurs in response to rectal distension (Wald and Tunuguntla, 1984).

Anal sensation

Perianal, anal and anal canal sensation are all impaired in the elderly and may also significantly contribute towards faecal incontinence when there is severe faecal loading (Read *et al.*, 1985; Barrett *et al.*, 1989). The combination of poor anal sensation and impaired ability to increase anal squeeze pressure voluntarily also increases the risk of faecal incontinence occurring when faecal material enters the anal canal.

The sampling reflex is an important component of the continence mechanism which has not yet been studied in elderly patients though impairment has been demonstrated in studies performed on younger patients (see p. 48).

Laxative induced faecal incontinence

Faecal incontinence may also be produced by the treatment of faecal impaction especially when problems with mobility prolong the time required to respond to the call to stool. Administration of laxatives, especially when a potent preparation is used, may therefore induce faecal incontinence.

Conclusion

Faecal soiling in faecally loaded patients is probably due to the combination of a number of factors which include an obtuse anorectal angle, low anal pressures, and alterations in anorectal sensation.

References

Barrett JA. (1988). A study of the anorectal pathophysiology of geriatric patients with faecal incontinence. MD thesis. University of Liverpool.

Barrett JA, Brocklehurst JC, Kiff ES, Ferguson G. (1989) Anal function in geriatric patients with faecal incontinence. *Gut*; **30**: 1244–51.

Barrett JA, Brocklehurst JC, Kiff ES, Ferguson G, Faragher EB. (1990) Rectal motility studies in geriatric patients with faecal incontinence. *Age and Ageing*; **19**: 311–17.

Barrett JA, Faragher EB, Kiff ES, Ferguson G, Brocklehurst JC. (1988) Why are geriatric patients incontinent of faeces? *Clin Sci*; **75**(Suppl 19): 10 P.

Brocklehurst JC. (1985) Colonic disease in the elderly. *Clin Gastroenterol*; **14**: 725–47.

Buser WD, Miner PB. (1986) Delayed rectal sensation with faecal incontinence. Successful treatment using anorectal manometry. *Gastroenterology*; **91**: 1186–91.

Ferguson GH, Redford J, Barrett JA, Kiff ES. (1989) The appreciation of rectal distension in faecal incontinence. *Dis Colon Rectum*; **32**: 964–7.

Read NW, Abouzekry L. (1986) Why do patients with faecal impaction have faecal incontinence. *Gut*; **27**: 283–7.

Read NW, Abouzekry L, Read MG, Howell P, Ottewell D, Donnelly TC. (1985) Anorectal function in elderly patients with faecal impaction. *Gastroenterology*; **89**: 959–66.

Rogers J, Levy DM, Henry MM, Misiewicz JJ. (1988) Pelvic floor neuropathy: a comparative study of diabetes mellitus and idiopathic faecal incontinence. *Gut*; **29**: 756–61.

Tobin GW, Brocklehurst JC. (1986) Faecal incontinence in residential homes for the elderly: prevalence, aetiology and management. *Age and Ageing*; **15**: 41–6.

Varma JS, Bradnock J, Smith RG, Smith AN. (1988). Constipation in the elderly. A physiologic study. Diseases of the Colon and Rectum. 31: 111–115.

Wald A, Tunuguntla AK. (1984) Anorectal sensorimotor dysfunction in faecal incontinence and diabetes mellitus. Modification with biofeedback therapy. *New Eng J Med*; **310**: 1282–87.

14

Faecal incontinence secondary to cerebral disease

Many of the mechanisms that maintain continence are reflex responses. The act of defaecation, however, does require a significant conscious effort. Loss of this input tends to lead quickly to faecal loading to an extent that will overcome the usual continence mechanisms. Diseases that affect cerebral function may therefore lead to faecal incontinence. These will be considered in this chapter under the following broad headings:

1. Impaired consciousness;
2. Patients with dementing illnesses;
3. Stroke;
4. Parkinson's disease.

Impaired consciousness

Faecal incontinence is inevitable in the unconscious patient unless preventive measures are taken and it is also well recognised in critically ill patients particularly when consciousness is impaired. An example of this is the incontinence that may occur in stroke victims which will be discussed later in this chapter.

Moderate or minor degrees of impaired consciousness, e.g. secondary to the use of sedative drugs, may also lead to faecal incontinence.

Patients with dementing illnesses

Faecal incontinence is very common in patients with dementing illnesses, e.g. Alzheimer's disease and multi-infarct disease. Barrett *et al.* (1990) included patients with dementing illnesses in their study performed in a department of Geriatric Medicine. Twenty-nine percent (59%) of the 49 faecally incontinent patients that they studied were considered to have clinical evidence of a dementing illness. This was significantly higher than the prevalence in the elderly control patients (5/31 (16%).

Incontinence in patients with dementing illnesses has been called neurogenic faecal incontinence by Brocklehurst (1985). Continued use of this term may, however, cause some difficulty as other groups use the term to describe anorectal incontinence or idiopathic faecal incontinence, though this would be more accurately described as a neuropathic disorder.

The main causes of faecal incontinence in patients with dementing illnesses are:

a) Loss of awareness;
b) Behavioural abnormalities;
    and possibly
c) Unstable rectum (uninhibited rectal contractions).

Loss of awareness

Patients with severe cognitive impairment can be expected to be less aware of rectal distension than non-demented patients. Barrett (1988) found that the mean volume of rectal balloon distension required to produce awareness of a 'call to stool' was 150mls in the 20 demented patients studied, compared with 99mls in the non-demented elderly patients studied (95% confidence interval of the difference between the means = 15–87mls). No difference however was found between the incontinent demented patients (mean 162mls. 95% CI = 104–221) and the continent demented patients studied (mean 134mls. 95% CI = 70–199).

Loss of awareness of the accumulation of faeces within the rectum tends to lead to gross faecal loading which ultimately leaks out in these patients who make no attempt to defaecate. Gross faecal loading was present in 73% of the incontinent demented patients studied by Barrett *et al.* (1990). Faecal leakage is uncommon in the absence of faecal loading.

Behavioural

Patients with dementing illnesses, however, do not all fit into the above category. Many retain their awareness of rectal distension and experience the 'call to stool' but unfortunately their response to this is to defaecate in inappropriate places, e.g. on the lounge carpet, on dining room chairs, in bed, etc. These patients may exhibit other behavioural disturbances, e.g. coprophagia, faecal smearing, inappropriate micturition, aggression, abusive language, etc. They pose a major problem to their carers and usually require institutional care unless the problem can be resolved.

It can be debated whether this is defined as incontinence but it does not alter the fact that the management of these patients is very difficult.

Unstable rectum (uninhibited rectal contractions)

Other explanations have been sought to explain the mechanism of faecal incontinence in patients with dementing illnesses. Animal studies suggest that there is some degree of cerebral control of rectal motility.

Garry (1933) found the rectum to be invariably inactive after decerebration in cats which he attributed to inhibitory impulses arising in the lumbosacral cord. Langworthy and Rosenberg (1939a) sectioned the brains of cats at different levels and assessed the rectal response to balloon distension. They found that after transection of the brain stem cephalic to the acoustic colliculi the rectum was hyperactive to stretch stimuli and that strong waves of contraction lead to expulsion of a distended balloon from the rectum. Contractions were not seen in response to distension following section of the brain through the medulla and the rectum was able to accommodate a larger volume than normal without expulsion of the balloon. A tonic mechanism in the mid brain controlling rectal smooth muscle was offered as the explanation for these observations (Langworthy and Rosenberg, (1939a; Denny-Brown and Robertson, 1935).

Langworthy and Rosenberg (1939b) also studied hemiplegic and paraplegic patients and found a response similar to that which followed transection of the brain stem cephalic to the acoustic colliculi. They suggested that the observed rectal hyperactivity was due to loss of normal inhibitory control exerted by the cerebral motor cortex.

Regular rectal contractions appear to be the normal rectal motility response to distension in young people whereas the normal rectal response in the elderly appears to be a flat motility trace with few if any rectal contractions (see p. 34). Barrett *et al.* (1990) elicited rectal contractions during rectal distension in 41% of their elderly control patients most of which occur either at the onset of rectal distension or soon afterwards (see Fig. 16, p. 34).

Approximately 10% of elderly control subjects exhibit regular or multiple rectal contractions (Barrett *et al.*, 1990; Read *et al.*, 1985) which is considerably lower than the incidence of 71% reported in young control patients (Read *et al.*, 1986). Prolonged recordings of rectal activity have not been performed in the elderly.

Rectal motility has also been assessed in elderly patients with global cerebral disease (Brocklehurst, 1951; Barrett *et al.*, 1990).

Brocklehurst (1951) performed balloon distension of the rectum up to a maximum of 250ml on 19 'senile' incontinent patients, many of whom were confused, and compared the response with that obtained in 11 continent elderly subjects. The control subjects were all able to retain the balloon to full inflation but seven (37%) of the incontinent patients expelled the balloon after 100–200mls of air had been instilled following a rectal contraction. These contractions developed during distension in the majority of the incontinent patients (13/19 (68%)) but in only one of the control subjects. Brocklehurst (1951) suggested that the higher incidence of rectal contractions in these patients was due to loss of cortical inhibition and that they resemble the detrusor contractions described in the 'uninhibited neurogenic bladder' (Brocklehurst and Dillane, 1966).

Barrett *et al.* (1990) compared the anorectal function of 34 patients with dementing illnesses with 61 non-demented patients, but demented patients with behavioural disturbances, e.g. aggression, were not studied for obvious reasons. They measured rectal motility both at rest and during rectal distension using two different devices one of which was used to simulate firm stool (an air filled party balloon). The soft stool model (a water filled condom which was used to perform proctometrograms) was involuntarily expelled more frequently by the incontinent patients (67%) than the firm stool model (18%) which suggests that faecal incontinence is more likely to occur when stool is soft in consistency.

Multiple rectal contractions during rectal distension were found more frequently in demented patients (40%) than in non-demented patients (11%). Loss of cortical inhibition therefore appears to lead to the development of uninhibited rectal contractions as previously suggested (Langworthy and Rosenberg, 1939a and 1939b; Brocklehurst, 1951). Similar uninhibited rectal contractions have also been demonstrated in patients with evidence of frontal lobe injury (Weber *et al.*, 1990). The incidence of multiple rectal contractions during rectal distension in elderly incontinent patients (25%), however, is not significantly different from that in elderly controls (11%) or in continent faecally loaded elderly patients (Barrett *et al.*, 1990).

Information from rectal saline infusion studies provides some insight into the mechanism(s) which lead to expulsion of faeces. Continence to the infusion of 1500mls of saline into the rectum is impaired in incontinent patients (Read *et al.*, 1979; Leigh and Turnberg, 1982; Matheson and Keighley, 1981).

Anorectal manometry performed by Read *et al.* (1983) during saline infusion into the rectum revealed that in normal subjects the rectal pressure never rose above anal pressure and leakage of saline did not occur. Leakage of saline in incontinent patients always coincided with a peak of rectal pressure which was greater than anal pressure. Leakage appeared to occur either because the internal sphincter was weak and easily inhibited or because peak rectal pressures were abnormally high due to strong rectal contractions.

It is tempting therefore to attribute faecal incontinence in demented geriatric patients to peaks of rectal pressure occurring with these uninhibited rectal contractions, as involuntary expulsion of the rectal balloons in the rectal distension studies is often preceded by a strong rectal contraction (Fig. 26) (Brocklehurst, 1951; Barrett *et al.*, 1990). No significant difference, however, has been found in the peak rectal pressures between either continent and incontinent patients with dementing illnesses or between continent and incontinent patients with faecal loading (Barrett, 1988). Anal resting pressure is, however, significantly reduced in the faecally incontinent demented patients.

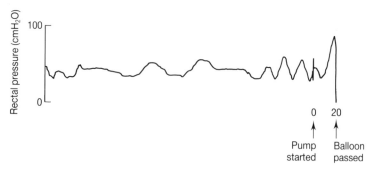

Fig. 26 Proctometrogram trace from an incontinent patient with advanced dementia demonstrating rectal contractions at rest which inrease in amplitude during rectal distension. (Reproduced from Barrett *et al., Age and Ageing*; 1990)

Barrett *et al*. (1990) also found a correlation between expulsion of the proctometrogram balloon (condom) and low anal resting pressure, low anal squeeze pressure, and the presence of rectal contractions on rectal distension. Expulsion of the party balloon, i.e. firm stool model, however, was only correlated with low anal resting pressure. It was not correlated with the presence of rectal contractions during rectal distension.

The lack of any difference between incontinent and continent individuals in the incidence of rectal contractions despite the increased incidence of rectal contractions in demented patients suggests that uninhibited rectal contractions do not play a major role in the overall mechanism of faecal incontinence. This is confirmed by the absence of a significant contribution by rectal contractions during rectal distension to the prediction of the presence of faecal incontinence in a mathematical model produced from this study (Barrett, 1988) (see also p. 126).

Faecal incontinence, even in demented patients, does not therefore appear to be solely due to unstable rectal contractions. The correlation between rectal contractions on rectal distension and passage of the condom suggests that rectal contractions may play a role in the passage of soft or liquid stool which may be similar to the passage of urine that follows unstable detrusor contractions but rectal contractions are unlikely to be responsible for the expulsion of firm stool.

The contribution of uninhibited rectal contractions to faecal incontinence is therefore small and insignificant. The state of contraction of the anal sphincters, however, appears to play an important role in the maintenance of continence in these patients, especially when the rectum is loaded with soft faeces.

The presence of a dementing illness has not been found to be associated with any significant change in anal resting pressure but anal squeeze pressures are lower than in control subjects (see Table 2). Full compliance with the measurement of squeeze pressure is not possible in all these patients which clearly contributes towards the observed differences.

If, however, low anal squeeze pressure is due to external anal sphincter weakness then this is unlikely to be due to pudendal neuropathy as the pudendal nerve terminal motor latency has been found to be normal in patients with dementing illnesses (Barrett, 1988).

Internal sphincter weakness is the most important anorectal factor leading to the development of faecal incontinence in demented patients. The anal resting pressure in the faecally incontinent demented patients is lower than in the continent demented patients (Barrett, 1988) (see Table 3).

There has been some interest in investigating the pathways between the rectum and the brain using electrical stimulation methods whilst recording evoked potentials.

Haldeman *et al.* (1982) reported successfully recording evoked potentials at the level of the L1 vertebra and at the Cz–2 EEG recording site following stimulation of the dorsal nerve of the penis or clitoris, a branch of the pudendal nerve.

Frieling *et al.* (1989) demonstrated that it is possible to record evoked potentials on the scalp after electrically stimulating the rectosigmoid. They examined eight patients and presented the averaged traces in their paper. These recordings, however, failed to demonstrate consistent intrasubject or intersubject patterns. Meunier (1990) questioned the safety of Frieling *et al.*'s technique of repeated electrical stimulation in the rectum in the presence of potentially inflammable gases.

Table 2 Comparison of anal sphincter pressures between elderly patients with a dementing illness and their non-demented controls. (Data from Barrett, 1988)

	Demented (n = 32)	Non-demented (n = 50)	p
Mean anal resting pressure (cmH$_2$0)	59	72	0.07
Mean anal squeeze pressure (cmH$_2$0)	31	50	0.05

Table 3 Comparison of anal sphincter pressures between continent and incontinent elderly patients with a dementing illness. (Data from Barrett, 1988)

	Demented, incontinent (n = 22)	Demented, not incontinent (n = 10)	p
Mean anal resting pressure (cmH$_2$0)	48	86	< 0.001
95% confidence interval for the difference bewteen the means = 20–56			
Median anal squeeze pressure (cmH$_2$0)	21	33	0.06
Range	0–129	10–104	

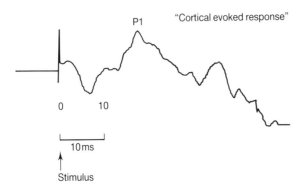

Fig. 27 'Cortical evoked potential' recorded from Cz–2cm electroencephalogram (EEG) electrode position following transrectal stimulation of the pudendal nerve. (Reproduced from Barrett, 1988)

Meunier suggested that endorectal mechanical stimulation produced by alternate rectal balloon distension and deflation could be a more relevant stimulus but he found large intersubject variability.

Barrett, Kiff and Ferguson performed pilot studies attempting to develop a method of measuring pudendal sensory and cortical evoked responses (Barrett, 1988). They stimulated the pudendal nerve using the transrectal device and equipment employed in the measurement of pudendal terminal motor latency.

They made cortical recordings from an active electrode placed in the midline of the scalp 2cm behind the Cz EEG recording site (Cz–2) determined by the international 10–20 electrode placement protocol. The reference electrode was placed in the midline of the forehead above the glabella (Epz) and an earth electrode was placed on the lateral aspect of the forehead. Five hundred averaged stimuli were administered to the pudendal nerve but this was uncomfortable due to anal contraction around the finger stall. An averaged response was recorded (Fig. 27). These revealed multiple positive and negative deflections but these were not consistent, unlike Haldeman *et al.*'s (1982) recordings.

They also attempted to record pudendal sensory evoked responses from an active electrode placed on the skin overlying the L2 vertebra. Approximately 500 stimuli were administered five times per second to the the pudendal nerve and the average of the responses was recorded (Fig. 28).

The response, however, did not appear to represent true sensory evoked potentials as it was also possible to record this response from sites other than over the spine, e.g. buttocks. The first peak of the response corresponded with the motor response peak measured from the external sphincter which suggested that these were motor responses rather than sensory evoked responses. The method was therefore abandoned.

Frieling *et al.*'s (1989) suggestion that these techniques may be useful in the study of patients with constipation and/or faecal incontinence is not supported by the current evidence.

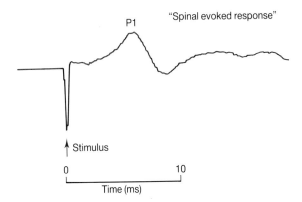

P1

"Spinal evoked response"

↑ Stimulus

0

10

Time (ms)

Fig. 28 'Spinal evoked potentials' recorded at the levelof the L1 vertebra following transrectal stimulation of the pudendal nerve. (Reproduced from Barrett, 1988)

Stroke

Bowel problems are very common in patients who have suffered a stroke and who have acquired significant disability. Impaired consciousness is the main cause of faecal incontinence in the early stages.

Brocklehurst *et al.* (1985) found that faecal incontinence occurred in 30% of stroke patients but was present in only two (3%) of the 62 survivors studied 12 months after the onset of their stroke. Fullerton (personal communication) confirmed these finding in his study of 205 stroke patients (Fullerton *et al.*, 1988). In a multivariate analysis he found the initial level of consciousness to be the most important factor predicting the development of faecal incontinence in the early stages. He also found that the patients who were incontinent of faeces six months after their stroke tended not to have been incontinent initially. Less than 10% of those who were initially incontinent were still incontinent after six months.

Data from the multicentre GUESS 2 study of 1500 stroke patients (Barer personal communication) demonstrates variability from 0–8% in the incidence of frequent faecal incontinence (at least one episode per week) at the time of discharge from the participating hospitals.

Constipation and/or faecal incontinence may affect stroke patients who have previously had normal bowel habit. Faecal loading is the main cause of faecal incontinence in conscious stroke patients. The factors that may contribute towards this include:

1. Poor mobility;
2. Poor oral intake of food/fluid especially when there is difficulty swallowing which occurs in 45% of stroke patients but resolves within two weeks in approximately 90% of these (Gordon *et al.*, 1987);

3. Inability to empty bowels. Psychological or other factors may prevent easy evacuation. Patients who are asked to defaecate on a bed pan or on a commode behind a thin screen with other patients, members of staff and/or visitors on the other side of the screen are likely to experience difficulty. They may be able to defaecate if they are given sufficient privacy when they are seated on a toilet or commode.

In the absence of constipation other problems in patients who have had severe strokes may lead to faecal incontinence. These include severe perceptual problems, cognitive problems, poor comprehension and/or speech problems. These may improve during the course of a rehabilitation programme.

Parkinson's disease

Constipation and gastrointestinal motility disorders are common in Parkinson's disease though the extent of the problem has not been formally investigated. Faceal incontinence may accompany the above problems or occur due to a chronic confusional state, e.g. Alzheimer's disease that often develops as Parkinson's disease progresses or vice versa.

References

Barrett JA. (1988) A study of the anorectal pathophysiology of geriatric patients with faecal incontinence. MD thesis. University of Liverpool.

Barrett JA, Brocklehurst JC, Kiff ES, Ferguson G, Faragher EB. (1990) Rectal motility studies in geriatric patients with faecal incontinence. *Age and Ageing*; **19**: 311–17.

Brocklehurst JC. (1951) *Incontinence in Old Age*. Livingstone, Edinburgh.

Brocklehurst JC. (1985) Colonic disease in the elderly. *Clin Gastroenterol*; **14**: 725–47.

Brocklehurst JC, Andrews K, Richards B, Laycock PJ. (1985) Incidence and correlates of incontinence in stroke patients. *J Am Geriat Soc*; **33**: 540–2.

Brocklehurst JC, Dillane JB. (1966) Studies of the female bladder in old age. *Gerontol Clin*; **8**: 306–19.

Denny-Brown DE, Robertson EG. (1935) An investigation of the nervous control of defaecation. *Brain*; **58**: 256–310.

Frieling T, Enck P, Wienbeck M. (1989) Cerebral responses evoked by electrical stimulation of rectosigmoid in normal subjects. *Dig Dis Sci*; **34**: 202–5.

Fullerton KJ, MacKenzie G, Stout RW. (1988) Prognostic indices in stroke. *Quart J Med*; **250**: 147–62.

Garry RC. (1933) The nervous control of the caudal region of the large bowel in the cat. *J Phys*; **77**: 422–31.

Gordon C, Langton Hewer R, Wade DT. (1987) Dysphagia in acute stroke. *Br Med J*; **295**: 411–14.

Haldeman S, Bradley WE, Bhatia NN, Johnson BK. (1982) Pudendal evoked responses. *Arch Neur*; **39**: 280–3.

Langworthy OR, Rosenberg SJ. (1939a) The control by the central nervous system of the rectal smooth muscle. *J Neur*; **2**: 356

Langworthy OR, Rosenberg SJ. (1939b) Abnormalities of rectal tone and contraction in paraplegia and hemiplegia. *Am J Dig Dis*; **6**: 455–8.

Leigh RJ, Turnberg LA. (1982) Faecal incontinence: the unvoiced symptom. *Lancet*; **i**: 1349–51.

Matheson DM, Keighley MRB. (1981) Manometric evaluation of rectal prolapse and faecal incontinence. *Gut*; **22**: 126–9.

Meunier PD. (1990) Endorectal cerebral evoked potentials. *Dig Dis Sci*; **35**: 539–41.

Read NW, Abouzekry L, Read MG, Howell P, Ottewell D, Donnelly TC. (1985) Anorectal function in elderly patients with faecal impaction. *Gastroenterology*; **89**: 959–66.

Read NW, Harford WV, Schmulen AC, Read MG, Santa Ana CA, Fordtran JS. (1979) A clinical study of patients with faecal incontinence and diarrhoea. *Gastroenterology*; **76**: 747–56.

Read NW, Haynes WG, Bartolo DCC, *et al.* (1983) Use of anorectal manometry during rectal infusion of saline to investigate sphincter function in incontinent patients. *Gastroenterology*; **85**: 105-13.

Read NW, Timms JM, Barfield LJ, Donnelly TC, Bannister JJ. (1986) Impairment of defaecation in young women with severe constipation. *Gastroenterology*; **90**: 53–60.

Weber J, Delangre T, Hannequin D, Beuret-Blanquart F, Denis P. Anorectal manometric anomalies in seven patients with frontal lobe brain damage. (1990) *Dig Dis Sci*; **35**: 225–30.

15

Faecal incontinence in the elderly – overview

The causes of faecal incontinence were classified on p. 70 as:

a) Immobility;
b) Symptomatic faecal incontinence;
c) Faecal incontinence secondary to constipation and faecal impaction;
d) Faecal incontinence secondary to cerebral disease:
    i. Impaired consciousness;
    ii. Patients with dementing illnesses.
    iii.Stroke.
    iv.Parkinson's disease.
e) Anorectal incontinence (idiopathic faecal incontinence);
    i. Anal sphincter and pelvic floor muscle weakness;
    ii. Anorectal sensory loss.

The multifactorial nature of faecal incontinence in the elderly is well recognised by clinicians. The relative contribution of the various factors to the overall problem of faecal incontinence in elderly disabled patients has been analysed in a multivariate analysis of the studies performed by Barrett (1988).

Results from anorectal studies performed on 49 faecally incontinent patients from a typical Department of Geriatric Medicine were included in the analysis. Most of these patients had been faecally incontinent for more than 12 months with the frequency of the episodes ranging between one per week and six per day. Sixty-nine percent were faecally loaded. A clinical diagnosis of a dementing illness was made in 59% of the incontinent patients. Only 16% of the 31 elderly control patients from the same department were considered demented. Eighty-four percent of the faecally incontinent patients were also incontinent of urine. Brocklehurst *et al*. (1977) have also shown that faecal incontinence associated with with a high incidence of bacteriuria. The elderly faecally incontinent patients were also found to be significantly less mobile than the elderly controls (see Table 4). Data from anorectal studies performed on 19 elderly patients with faecal loading without faecal incontinence and from studies on 57 younger control subjects recruited from the surgical department was also included in the analysis.

Stepwise forward multiple regression analysis was performed to determine as far as possible which variables were related to the frequency of faecal incontinence. Significance was set at the 10% level. The initial analysis was based on the 35 patients who had all the variables measured. It revealed that the frequency of faecal incontinence was related to anal resting pressure, mobility and the presence of reflex contraction of the external anal sphincter in response to rectal distension. These combined contributed 34% of the variance in the mathematical model devised by the analysis.

A further stepwise forward analysis was performed on 81 cases by substituting the median value for each variable where data was missing. These cases were all geriatric patients as the surgical patients did not have rectal motility studies. The frequency of faecal incontinence on this analysis was found to be strongly associated with anal resting pressure. The presence of faecal loading was the only other factor

Table 4 Comparison of the characteristics of elderly patients with faecal incontinence, elderly patients with faecal loading without incontinence and elderly and younger control subjects with normal bowel habit. (Data from Barrett *et al.*, 1989)

	Elderly faecal incontinence (n = 47)	Elderly faecel loading (n = 19)	Elderly controls (n = 31)	Younger controls (n = 57)
Female	63%	63%	71%	40%
Mean age (years)	80.3	75.8	76.5	47.5
Faecal loading	34 (69%)	19 (100%)	0	0
Urinary incontinence	41 (84%)	9 (47%)	5 (16%)	0
Dementia*	26 (59%)	6 (33%)	5 (16%)	0
Mental status score (median)	4.5	9.7	9.8	10
Other neurological disease	21 (43%)	10 (53%)	11 (36%)	0
Diabetes	2 (4%)	3 (16%)	6 (19%)	0
Mobility				p < 0.001 Corrected chi-squared
Walks without aids or assistance	18%	16%	19%	100%
Walks with aids or assistance	18%	60%	68%	0
Immobile	64%	26%	13%	0

* = The prevalence of dementia was highest amongst the faecally incontinent patients. The patients with faecal incontinence had lower mental status scores than patients in the other groups (Kruskal Wallis one way analysis of variance, p < 0.001).

related to the frequency of incontinence. Thirty-five percent of the variance was accounted for.

A discriminant analysis was also performed to determine which factors predicted the presence of faecal incontinence. The significant factors determined by this analysis were mobility, age, faecal loading and anal resting pressure.

The residual variance unaccounted for after each step of the procedure is given below:

	Residual variance
Mobility score (m)	82%
Age (a)	75%
Faecal impaction score (f)	71%
Anal resting pressure (r)	65%

The equation produced by this discriminant analysis accounted for 35% of the variance. The equation was then used to produce a discriminant score for each patient:

Discriminant score =

$$4.46 - (0.55 \times m) - (0.05 \times a) - (0.65 \times f) + (0.02 \times r)$$

A negative score predicted that an individual would be incontinent. A positive score predicted normal continence. The conclusion from the discriminant score calculated for each patient included in the study was compared with each patients actual faecal continence. The discriminant score correctly predicted continence/incontinence in 132 (85%) of the 156 cases. Fourteen (29%) of the incontinent patients and ten (9%) of the continent patients were assigned to the incorrect group. There was thus a tendency of the scores to underestimate the presence of faecal incontinence.

The scores are plotted in Fig. 29. It will be noted that among the continent patients there are two peaks. The first peak corresponds to the geriatric department patients and the second peak to the younger surgical department control patients (see Fig. 30). The continence of all the surgical patients was correctly predicted. Exclusion of the surgical patients from the analysis of the scores reduces the predictive accuracy of the calculated scores to 76%.

The factors that were included in these multivariate analyses that did not significantly contribute to either the frequency or the presence of faecal incontinence were rectal contractions, rectal sensation and mental status score.

The results of the multivariate analysis do not, however, account for all the variance probably because some important variables are either unknown or were not measured, e.g. the anorectal angle.

Frequent or continuous leakage of faeces in elderly patients who are faecally incontinent due to faecal loading appears to be due to internal anal sphincter weakness whereas younger patients with anorectal incontinence tend to experience severe urgency and have a limited ability to prevent the involuntary expulsion of faeces due to external sphincter weakness.

It would appear from the discriminant analysis that the risk of an elderly person developing faecal incontinence is highest if he or she is immobile, old, and faecally loaded with a low anal resting pressure. Pudendal neuropathy and uninhibited rectal contractions do not play a significant role in causing faecal incontinence in the elderly though the expulsion of faeces may be preceded by rectal contraction(s). Inability

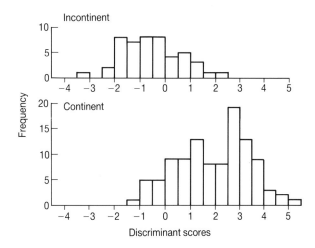

Fig. 29 Histogram of the discriminant scores calculated for elderly patients studied by Barrett (1988). Negative scores predicted the presence of faecal incontinence and positive scores normal continence. (Reproduced from Barrett, 1988)

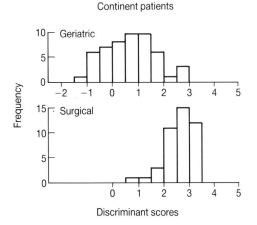

Fig. 30 Histograms of the discriminant scores calculated for the continent patients included in Barrett's (1988) study. Positive scores predict normal continence. The scores for the elderly control patients recruited from the surgical department are plotted separately. (Reproduced from Barrett, 1988)

of the internal sphincter to prevent this expulsion appears to be the most important factor leading to incontinence in these patients.

Barrett (1988) did not find a low mental status score to be among the variables predicting the presence of faecal incontinence in elderly patients. They may, however, have been a different result if the sample had been a random sample of the population which this study was not intended to be. It appears, however, that faecal incontinence in most demented patients is due to either faecal loading, low anal resting pressure or inhibition of the anal sphincter occurring before they are aware of rectal distension (Barrett, 1988).

References

Barrett JA. (1988) A study of the anorectal pathophysiology of geriatric patients with faecal incontinence. MD thesis. University of Liverpool.

Barrett JA, Brocklehurst JC, Kliff ES, Ferguson G, Fragher EB. (1989) Anal function in geriatric patients with faecal incontinence. *Gut*; **30**: 1244–51.

Brocklehurst JC, Bee P, Jones D, Palmer MK. (1977) Bacteriuria in geriatric hospital patients: its correlates and management. *Age and Ageing*. **6**: 240–5.

16

Clinical assessment of the faecally incontinent elderly patient

Faecal incontinence and/or constipation are problems that many patients are reluctant to discuss and for which thay are reluctant to seek help. Patients often consult their doctor about diarrhoea when the problem is actually faecal incontinence. Many patients manage to conceal their faecal incontinence for long periods (Read *et al.*, 1979; Leigh and Turnberg 1982; Drossman *et al.*, 1986). It is advisable therefore to ensure that patients who present complaining of diarrhoea are using the term correctly. Most incontinent patients will discuss their problem when asked they are asked direct questions about it.

The clinical assessment of the incontinent and/or constipated patient should include taking a thorough history and performing a physical examination which must include a rectal examination.

The history

The history taken should include an enquiry about the following:

1. Incontinence   — faecal
                        — Urinary
2. Onset of constipation (? acute or chronic)
3. Defaecation history
       Frequency of defaecation
       Stool consistency (hard/firm/soft stool)
       Straining on defaecation
       Rectal sensation (call to stool)

Can defaecation be delayed once the call to stool has been sensed?
Anorectal discomfort
Rectal prolapse
4.   Rectal bleeding
5.   Fluid and dietary intake
6.   Medications, especially constipating drugs and laxatives
7.   Obstetric history
No. of children
? Long labours
? Forceps delivery
? Perineal tears
8.   Anorectal surgery or hysterectomy

Patients with severe constipation should also be asked the following question; 'Some people with this problem use their fingers to assist the bowels to empty. Have you ever needed to do this?'

Physical examination

Physical examination of the constipated and/or faecally incontinent patient should include the following:

1.   General assessment of   — mobility
— hydration
— mental status (e.g. mental test score)
— general behaviour
— mood.
2.   Abdominal examination which should include careful palpation to detect the presence of any abdominal masses especially in the sigmoid colon.
3.   Digital anorectal examination, including observation for the presence of
— perineal descent
— faecal soiling
— haemorrhoids
— anal lesions e.g. fissure
— anal scars e.g. previous surgery
— gaping anus.

Perineal descent is a sign of pelvic floor muscle weakness. It can be considered present if the anus is at the level of or below the level of the ischial tuberosities of the pelvis either at rest or on attempted straining. The latter may also reveal the presence of rectal prolapse.
4.   Palpation — anal resting tone
— ability to squeeze anus tightly shut (good assessment of external anal sphincter and pelvic floor muscles).
— faecal loading (note stool consistency)
— rectal lesions, e.g. carcinoma, polyp.

Felt Bersma *et al.* (1988) have confirmed that it is possible at the bedside to obtain an indication of anal pressure despite previous comments to the contrary. In their study they compared estimates of anorectal pressures from digital palpation in 280 consecutive patients with anorectal manometry findings. They found a significant correlation between the palpation estimates and the measured values (Figs. 31 and 32).

Investigations.

These may include:

Biochemical profile – especially serum potassium, calcium;
Full blood count – especially haemoglobin;
Faecal occult bloods – when microscopic blood loss is suspected;
Thyroid function tests;
Abdominal radiograph;
    and/or
Sigmoidoscopy, barium enema, colonoscopy when a colorectal lesion(s) is suspected.

There are differing opinions concerning the performance of abdominal radiographs in constipated elderly patients. Smith and Lewis (1990) following their study, advocated that abdominal radiographs were

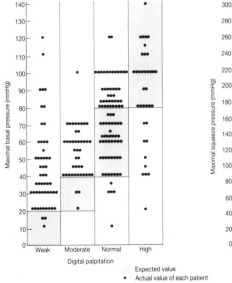
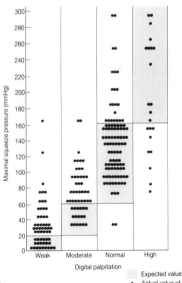

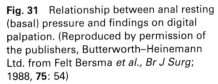

Fig. 31 Relationship between anal resting (basal) pressure and findings on digital palpation. (Reproduced by permission of the publishers, Butterworth–Heinemann Ltd. from Felt Bersma *et al.*, *Br J Surg*; 1988, **75**: 54)

Fig. 32 Relationship between anal squeeze pressure and findings on digital palpation. (Reproduced by permission of the publishers, Butterworth–Heinemann Ltd. from Felt Bersma *et al.*, *Br J Surg*; 1988, **75**: 54)

routinely performed as part of patient assessment to enable accurate detection of large bowel faecal loading. In their study they performed a digital rectal examination and abdominal radiograph on 101 consecutive patients admitted to a geriatric medical assessment unit. They found that 47% of their subjects had faecal loading of the rectum with soft faeces. Patients with large amounts of faeces in the rectum did not necessarily have radiographic evidence of colonic faecal loading and vice versa.

Perhaps, therefore, that study should be interpreted in a slightly different way because if a patient is found to have faecal loading on digital rectal examination then it is unlikely that the information from an abdominal radiograph is going to significantly influence his or her management. If, however, a patient presents with a history suggestive of constipation but the rectum is empty then a radiograph would be helpful in the detection of high faecal loading or to exclude intestinal obstruction when abdominal pain is a prominent feature.

Faecal incontinence may have a profound psychological effect on individual patients. This is discussed in Chapter 23.

References

Drossman DA, Sandler RS, Broom CM, McKee DC. (1986) Urgency and faecal soiling in people with bowel dysfunction. *Dig Dis Sci*; **31**: 1221–25.

Felt Bersma RJF, Klinkenberg-Knol EC, Meuwissen SGM. (1988) Investigation of anorectal function. *Br J Surg*; **75**: 53–5.

Leigh RJ, Turnberg LA. (1982) Faecal incontinence: the unvoiced symptom. *Lancet*; **i**: 1349–51.

Read NW, Harford WV, Schmulen AC, Read MG, Santa Ana CA, Fordtran JS. (1979) A clinical study of patients with faecal incontinence and diarrhoea. *Gastroenterology*; **76**: 747–56.

Smith RG, Lewis S. (1990) THe relationship between digital rectal examination and abdominal radiographs in elderly patients. *Age and Ageing*; **19**: 142–4.

17

Treatment of faecal incontinence – introduction

Improved understanding of the pathophysiology of faecal incontinence should be used to improve the treatment of patients with faecal incontinence.

Tobin and Brocklehurst (1986), in their study of incontinence in residential homes demonstrated that faecal incontinence in the elderly

Table 5 Results from Tobin and Brocklehurst's (1986) study of the use of simple treatment measures in the management of faecal incontinence. The results are split into three sections: (a) all incontinent patients, divided into the study group who were recommended for the active treatment and their controls; (b) the study group from (a) without the patients who did not actually receive the treatment compared with the control group; (c) the treatment results for patients primarily incontinent because of either faecal impaction or a dementing illness.

Outcome	Groups	
a) *All patients*	*Study*	*Control*
No longer incontinent	60%	32%
Incontinent < once per week	4%	14%
Incontinent > once per week	36%	54%
b) *Full compliance obtained*	*Study*	*Control*
No longer incontinent	87%	32%
Incontinent < once per week	3%	14%
Incontinent > once per week	10%	54%
c) *Full compliance obtained*	*Impaction*	*Dementia*
No longer incontinent	94%	75%
Incontinent < once per week	0	8%
Incontinent > once per week	6%	17%

is a treatable and preventable condition. When full compliance was achieved, simple therapeutic measures lead to complete resolution of faecal incontinence in 87% of their treatment group compared with 32% resolution in their control group (see Table 5).

In the elderly, faecal incontinence tends to be multifactorial in aetiology with considerable overlap between the main causes of faecal incontinence which have been described in the preceding chapters. In the following discussion of the treatment of faecal incontinence each of the main causes will be discussed separately in Chapters 18–21. The management of intractable faecal incontinence is discussed in Chapter 22 and psychological management in Chapter 23.

References

Tobin GW, Brocklehurst JC. (1986) Faecal incontinence in residential homes for the elderly: prevalence, aetiology and management. *Age and Ageing*; **15**: 41–46.

18

Treatment of faecal incontinence secondary to faecal loading

Faecal loading is the main cause of faecal incontinence in the elderly even in patients with dementia. A protocol for the management of faecal loading with or without faecal incontinence is summarised in the flow chart in Fig. 33.

Initial treatment of the incontinent faecally loaded patient

The initial aim in the treatment of the incontinent faecally loaded patient is to empty the rectum and colon.

Laxatives such as lactulose or stool softeners such as docusate (dioctyl sodium sulphosuccinate) are often prescribed first but this tends to be unsuccessful because many of these patients are loaded with very soft stool. Further softening tends to increase the frequency of incontinent episodes.

It is generally accepted that these patients are best managed by emptying the rectum from below by administering an enema each day until the faecal mass is cleared. Phosphate enemas which contain 10% sodium acid phosphate and 8% sodium phosphate in a total volume of 128mls are commonly used. The osmotic activity of sodium acid phosphate, which is poorly absorbed from the rectum, increases the water content of the stool. The rectal distension that follows probably induces defaecation by stimulating rectal motility.

Phosphate enemas are occasionally ineffective usually because the enema is not retained. In these patients a better result may be obtained with the use of a micro-enema or suppository. Micro-enemas (e.g. Micralax) contain agents which allow water to penetrate into and soften faeces and then stimulate defaecation, usually within 5–15 minutes.

Micro-enemas now tend to be used as the first choice agent rather than phosphate enemas because there have been case reports attributing serious local complications, e.g. rectal gangrene, to injury caused by the nozzle of the phosphate enema (Smith *et al.*, 1987; Sweeney *et al.*, 1986). If a phosphate enema is used then the nozzle of the enema should be pointed towards the posterior rectal wall. Enemas or suppositories

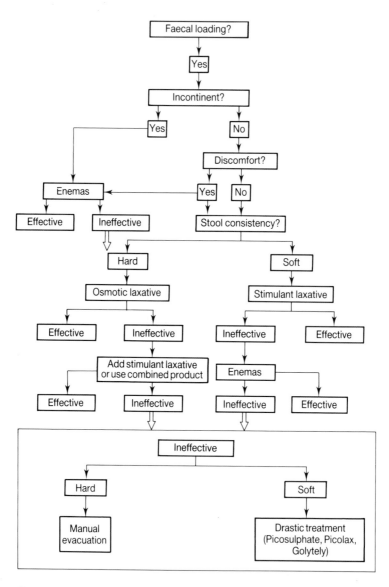

Fig. 33 Flow chart describing a simplified scheme for the management of faecal loading in elderly and/or disabled patients. (Reproduced from Barrett, *Geriatric Medicine Supplement*; March 1989, pp 14–18

often need to be given daily for 7–14 days to clear the bowel in patients with severe faecal loading.

Enemas and suppositories have been used for many years in the management of defaecatory problems. The current torpedo shape of suppositories dates back to a proposal from Henry S. Wellcome (1893). Abd-el-Maeboud *et al.* (1991) have recently reviewed their use. In their study performed in Cairo, they found that all but two of the 360 lay subjects and 260 medical personnel that they questioned considered that the commonsense method of insertion of the suppository with the apex foremost was the correct mode of insertion. Commonsense was cited as the evidence to support this practice in 86% of the study group.

In another part of their study they compared the two possible methods of suppository insertion, i.e. apex foremost or base foremost. They found that retention of the suppository in their 100 subjects was more easily achieved by inserting the base foremost in 98% of their subjects with no need to insert a finger into the anal canal (1% *v* 83%) and lower expulsion rates (0% *v.* 3%). Clearly therefore suppositories should be inserted with the base foremost. It is probable that the reverse gradient of pressure in the anal canal accounts for this phenomenon (Fig. 34).

Treatment of faecal loading which fails to respond to initial treatment

Standard treatment with enemas or suppositories is usually effective but there are some patients who require other methods to clear their bowels. Manual removal of faeces may be required for patients who are loaded with very hard faeces or for patients with an atonic rectum which cannot be emptied in any other way. This problem is particularly prevalent among patients with severe spinal cord lesions in whom the stimulatory nerve supply to the rectum (parasympathetic from the S 3, 4, 5 nerve roots) is deficient.

Very potent orally administered regimens to produce bowel clearance in one procedure have also been described.

Whole gut irrigation has been used for this purpose. Isotonic saline was infused into the stomach via a nasogastric tube at a rate of 2.5–3 litres per hour until the effluent emerging from the rectum was clear (Smith *et al.*, 1978). This procedure has now been abandoned as it may cause fatal water and sodium retention in the elderly. The risk of electrolyte disturbance and water retention is reduced by substituting mannitol for saline in the above regimen (Palmer and Khan, 1979; Davis *et al.*, 1980). A further modification of this regimen has been made with the substitution of polyethylene glycol for mannitol to produce 'Golytely' (Davis *et al.*, 1980). Puxty and Fox (1986) suggest this is a well tolerated effective treatment for faecal impaction in geriatric patients. The disadvantage, however, is that patients have to drink approximately ½ litre of Golytely to obtain the result.

Picolax ia an alternative preparation that may be used to clear the bowel. Picolax is a mixture of sodium picosulphate (a stimulant laxative) with citric acid and magnesium oxide (which form magnesium citrate in solution). Magnesium citrate is a poorly absorbed osmotic laxative which produces a semi-fluid or watery evacuation after 3–6 hours. Sodium picosulphate exerts its effect 10–14 hours after administration.

Picolax is used by many radiologists for bowel preparation prior to barium enema examination. It has been shown to produce an excellent bowel clearance and is better tolerated than mannitol as it causes less nausea and vomiting (Foord *et al.*, 1983). It has not, however, been compared with Golytely.

There is no doubt that Picolax is a potent laxative but its effects are unfortunately difficult to control when it is used in frail elderly patients with severe faecal loading. Very severe faecal incontinence may be produced in the 24 hours after administration. This can, however, be successfully contained in co-operative patients by using a faecal collection device (see p. 170).

Picolax or Golytely should be reserved for the treatment of severe faecal loading in patients who are resistant to conventional treatment, i.e. enemas. When Picolax is used the starting dose should be just ¼ of the manufacturer's recommended dose, i.e. ½ sachet as a single dose. If this is ineffective the dose can then be increased.

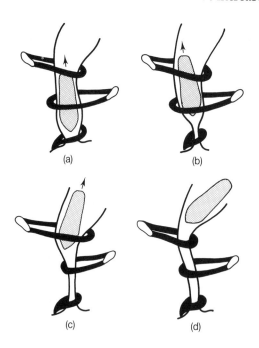

(a) suppository lies within relaxed external sphincter; (b) base loop contraction and intermediate loop relaxation; (c) intermediate loop contraction and top loop relaxation; (d) top loop contraction.

Fig. 34 A series of diagrams to demonstrate the action of the sphincter muscles after the introduction of a suppository into the anal canal 'blunt end first' and the subsequent reverse contractions which help its passage into the rectum. (Reproduced from Abd-el-Maeboud *et al.*, 1991)

For patients with faecal loading with soft stool use of sodium picosulphate alone without the magnesium citrate component of Picolax is also an effective potent laxative that appears to be less likely to produce uncontrollable bowel evacuation. The starting dose in these patients is 5mg given as a single dose but increased as required until bowel clearance is achieved. Some patients may need 40mg on alternate nights to stimulate defaecation.

Prevention of recurrence

Constipation with or without faecal incontinence is a very common feature of acute disabling ilnesses in the elderly, particularly in patients who have problems with their mobility. No data is currently available about the frequency of this problem or about the percentage of these patients whose bowel function returns to normal once they recover from their illness. Patients who do not recover completely may experience a continuing tendency to constipation. This probably accounts for Brocklehurst *et al.*'s (1983) observation that whole gut transit time does not necessarily change following the clearance of faecal masses from patients with severe faecal loading in continuing care wards for the elderly. The cause of this continuing tendency to constipation is unknown; immobility is clearly one important factor but other factors, e.g. the presence of a defaecatory abnormality, cannot be excluded.

A number of medical treatments are available to assist in the prevention of recurrent constipation. These will be discussed later.

The effect of an exercise programme followed by abdominal massage was studied by Resende (1989) in 12 elderly constipated patients who were residents in a hospital continuing care ward because of their disabilities. All 12 patients were immobile and had been on laxatives and/or enemas for at least six months. Whole gut transit times were markedly prolonged at entry to the study. Bowel medication was discontinued at that time but provision was made for this to be recommenced if required. If no bowel movement occurred for five days an enema was given.

During a 12 week treatment phase each patient had an exercise programme supervised by a physiotherapist on his or her bed for 20 minutes per day followed by a ten minute abdominal massage. The abdominal massage, however, did not appear to be very well tolerated as half of the patients found it to be either an unpleasant experience or refused it completely.

At the conclusion of the study whole gut transit times were unaltered. The number of days on which bowel movements occurred increased (pre-treatment 32%, during treatment 41%), and there was a reduction in the percentage of days during which faecal incontinence occurred (pre-treatment 7.5%, during treatment 3.4%). The percentage of days on which enemas were given fell from 9% before treatment to 3% on treatment and the number of days on which laxatives were given fell from 94% to 0.09%. Interpretation of these results is, however, difficult as laxative use was discouraged as part of the study and others have shown that education of staff (Julien *et al.*, 1983), carers and patients (Elazarion *et al.*, 1980) can lead to a major reduction in laxative use in elderly continuing care patients. Most of these patients did not require any laxatives in the six months following the study.

The exercise and massage programme may have been responsible for the changes observed as improved mobility during a rehabilitation treatment programme often leads to an improvement in bowel function in elderly patients with disabilities. The relative contributions made by the bed exercises and the massage is unknown. The evidence is not convincing enough to support any major change in the management of these patients apart from increasing physicians' awareness of the prospects of withdrawing laxative treatment from these patients without adverse effects.

Fibre and constipation

A high fibre diet has become popular in the management of lower gastro-intestinal problems easpecially constipation and diverticular disease. It is usually given as added bran but many people find this unpalatable and may experience flatulence and abdominal distension. These symptoms often prevent sufficient bran being taken to alter colonic function (Edwards *et al.*, 1988).

It is not clear how fibre alters gut function but it is interesting to note that Tomlin and Read (1988) found that the ingestion of plastic particles could also influence bowel function by reducing transit time, leading to a bulkier stool being produced. The effects of bran appear to be more marked with coarse bran than with fine processed bran.

There are also a number of bulking agents available as alternatives to bran. These include Isphagula (marketed in the preparations Fybogel, Isogel, Metamucil and Regulan), Sterculia and Methylcellulose.

Methylcellulose in normal healthy subjects leads to an increase in stool weight and faecal frequency (Hamilton *et al.*, 1988). In the same study of young chronically constipated patients (mean age 28 years) stool frequency, water content and faecal solids were all increased. There were no incontinent episodes reported but studies in the elderly have produced different results.

The effects of wheat bran in constipated patients have been reviewed by Muller-Lissner (1988) following a meta-analysis performed on the results of 20 studies of the use of bran either in volunteers, patients with irritable bowel syndrome, diverticular disease or constipation. Bran was found to be only partially effective in restoring the stool weight and gastrointestinal transit times of constipated patients to normal. High dietary fibre intake has also been shown to be associated with colonic faecal loading in immobile elderly patients (Donald *et al.*, 1985).

Andersson *et al.* (1979) studied ten patients from a Swedish geriatric unit and found that their whole gut mean transit time during treatment with a bulk laxative was 126 hours compared with 89 hours during treatment with bran. They advocated the use of bran on the basis of these results but admit in their discussion that many of their patients experienced faecal soiling during this treatment.

Ardron and Main (1990) studied the use of bran in 20 elderly immobile patients in a geriatric medical unit. They told the patients and staff that they were assessing the effects of the addition of fibre to the diet. In the study they gave placebo treatment, e.g. thickened soup for the first two weeks followed by four weeks treatment with 10g of bran/day and finally a three week placebo period similar to the first two weeks. During the treatment period there was an increase in stool weight and a reduction in the number of days on which stool was not passed. Ten of the 20 patients, however, became incontinent of faeces on the treatment compared with just three of the 20 being incontinent during the placebo phases.

Clarke and Scott (1976) also found faecal incontinence to be a problem in their elderly patients treated with bran.

In young patients or healthy mobile elderly people it is probably reasonable to encourage a high fibre intake as part of their normal diet in an attempt to reduce the risks of diverticular disease and to produce a bulkier softer stool to enable defaecation to proceed more easily. Elderly patients with faecal loading tend to already have soft bulky stools which have a tendency to leak when they are too loose in consistency as occurs when there is a high dietary fibre intake. The evidence about the risks of faecal incontinence occurring when bran is used in the treatment of constipation suggest that it should be avoided in elderly patients especially if they have mobility problems.

The general advice given to people in Western society to increase their fibre intake is based on the belief that high fibre intake accounts for the low incidence of diverticular disease in Africa (Burkitt *et al.*, 1972), It has been generally extrapolated from this observation that high fibre intake will benefit all people in Western society including the frail elderly despite the lack of any studies looking at this particular question.

Many hospitals and care homes therefore have a 'healthy eating' policy which includes the addition of fibre to the diet. They genuinely believe that this is benefiting their patients. The studies cited above suggest they should review this policy as it is more likely to cause faecal incontinence than any other measure.

Incontinent faecally loaded patients in these establishments can often have their continence restored by the simple measure of removing the added fibre from their diet. Nursing homes for the elderly should therefore be discouraged from adopting a 'high fibre diet for all residents' policy.

Laxatives

The main alternative to fibre is to use a laxative. The choice of a laxative should always be guided by the character of the stool and the patient's ability to defaecate.

In patients with hard stool it is better to use an osmotic laxative, e.g. lactulose, which is a synthetic disaccharide that is not digested or absorbed by the small intestine. It starts to exert its osmotic effect in the small bowel and is metabolised in the colon to short chain organic acids which are absorbed. The osmotic effect therefore does not continue throughout the colon. Lactulose significantly increases faecal weight, volume, water, and bowel movements (Bass and Dennis, 1981) and acts within two days. It is effective in the treatment of constipation (Wesselius-DeCasparis *et al.*, 1968) but it is expensive and many patients dislike the taste.

Faecal softeners, e.g. docusate sodium, act by lowering the surface tension of faeces and allowing the penetration of water. Docusate may also have a weak stimulatory effect but it is a poor laxative (Goodman *et al.*, 1976).

In patients with soft or formed stool a stimulant laxative is preferred. The most commonly used are senna (Senokot), sodium picosulphate and bisacodyl. These stimulant laxatives are best given at night to avoid faecal incontinence (Harvard and Hughes-Roberts, 1962).

Senna is an anthracine laxative which is hydrolysed, probably by bacteria in the colon (Hardcastle and Wilkins, 1970). Its derivatives are absorbed in the colon where they have a direct stimulatory effect on the myenteric plexus. Most patients respond to between 15 and 60mg daily (Marcus and Heaton, 1968). The laxative effect of sodium picosulphate is similar to senna (MacLennan and Pooler, 1975). Bisacodyl exerts its stimulant effect directly on the myenteric plexus (Hardcastle and Mann, 1968). It is not absorbed from the gut. It may be given orally or by suppository; defaecation usually occurs 35 to 75 minutes after the insertion of a suppository (Deiling *et al.*, 1959) or 10–12 hours after an oral dose.

Long term use of senna may produce melanosis coli and is also associated with myenteric degeneration (see p. 89). Ideally it should only be used for a short period of time but there are many patients who need a stimulant laxative on a long term basis to enable defaecation to proceed.

Codanthrusate, a combination of a stimulant (danthron) and a stool softener (docusate), offers an alternative choice especially for opiate induced constipation.

Danthromer, another combined laxative (danthron plus poloxamer), was a very popular laxative until its safety was questioned following a series of animal studies. Mori *et al.*, (1985) found caecal or colonic adenomas or adenocarcinomas in a number of rats treated with danthron 1500mg/kg/day for 16 months, which far exceeds the doses used in clinical practice. Only 12 of the original 18 rats survived 16 months which suggests that the dose used was too high for a valid carcinogenicity study. In a subsequent study of mice treated with 800mg/kg/day, hyperplastic changes were noted in the caecum and/or colon and liver adenomas were found in some treated and control animals (Mori *et al.*, 1986) and four treated animals developed liver carcinoma but this result has not been considered statistically significant (Twycross, 1989).

There is great doubt about the relevance of these animal studies as other studies have not produced any evidence of danthron being a tumour promoter (Brown, 1980). No case of unexpected caecal, colonic or liver neoplasia has been reported from autopsies of patients treated with danthron containing laxatives.

The most popular danthromer preparation, Dorbanex, was withdrawn from the market after these reports, It is now available again as Codalax and is licensed for use in the management of constipation in the elderly and the terminally ill.

Liquid paraffin, once a popular laxative, should not be used as it may cause a lipoid pneumonia if inhaled.

The prokinetic agent cisapride may become an alternative to laxative treatment in the future though at present its cost rather prevents its widespread use in constipation. The effect of cisapride on upper gastro-intestinal function is well recognised and data is now available about its effect on large bowel function.

Cisapride 10mg orally has been shown, using scintigraphic techniques in six normal subjects to reduce the half life of transit through the colon from 38.5 to 11.1 hours with the effects being most marked in the ascending and transverse colon (Krevsky *et al.*, 1987; Lederer *et al.*, 1986). In patients with delayed colonic transit the half emptying time of the caecum and ascending colon were also significantly reduced after cisapride (Krevsky *et al.*, 1987).

Madsen (1990), however, reported that normal subjects on the fifth day of treatment with cisapride 10mg four times daily exhibit a delay in large bowel transit despite more rapid gastric emptying and reduced small bowel transit times.

Muller-Lissner *et al.* (1987) have demonstrated that the use of cisapride 20mg bd for 8–12 weeks in patients with chronic constipation progressively increases stool frequency and the number of stools of normal consistency whilst reducing laxative intake. These effects develop gradually over a number of weeks and begin to produce significant benefit compared with placebo effects during the 5th–8th week of treatment. When treatment was discontinued at the end of the study the effects continued for at least four weeks after active treatment ceased. The optimum duration of treatment is unknown.

There has also been some experience in the use of cisapride in the treatment of chronic constipation in patients with paraplegia due to severe spinal injuries (Binnie *et al.*, 1988). Their mean colonic transit time was reduced from 185 to 123 hours with cisapride 10mg tds. They also found that maximal rectal capacity was reduced from 306mls to 224mls and there was a significant reduction in residual urine volume from 52mls to 28mls. One of the ten patients in this study went into urinary retention after the drug was suddenly withdrawn. No changes were seen in routine biochemistry including urea and electrolytes. The long term effects of cisapride in these patients has not yet been reported.

How effective are laxatives at preventing constipation and faecal incontinence?

Laxatives are administered to many elderly disabled patients to prevent recurrent constipation. Brocklehurst *et al.* (1983), however, found in a study of patients in long stay geriatric wards that neither lactulose or Dorbanex (danthromer) prevented constipation recurring, although they were better than no treatment. Many of these patients required regular emptying of their bowel from below using either enemas (preferably micro-enemas) or suppositories (Glycerine or bisacodyl). It is more likely that these will be needed in patients who continue to have a tendency to faecal incontinence due to their persistent faecal loading.

Some insight into the factors which determine the outcome of the treatment of chronic constipation and overflow incontinence has been evaluated in two studies in children. Loening-Baucke (1989) studied 97 children (mean age 9.0 years) and found that 43% had recovered after one year of a combination of milk of magnesia, high fibre diet and bowel training. The children who did not recover were more likely to have originally had frequent soiling episodes, more severe constipation and were less likely to be able to defaecate simulated stools. Recovery was not found to be related to behavioural group.

Nolan *et al.* (1991) studied 169 children with combined constipation and faecal incontinence (encopresis). They compared laxative treatment (initially three enemas followed by oral laxatives) in combination with a behavioural modification programme designed to promote regular toileting with regular toileting alone. They found that improvement was more likely with the combined treatment. Fifty-one percent of the children were continent after 12 months compared with only 36% of the patients in the behavioural treatment group.

In the past soap and water enemas had a major role in the treatment of constipation but their use has declined now to the extent that the procedure is rarely performed. There are, however, a small number of patients who are reluctant to accept any alternative treatment as they have become accustomed to having their bowels cleared with this regimen. Occasionally a new patient may need a soap and water enema when other treatment has failed.

Biofeedback in the treatment of constipation

This will be discussed in Chapters 21 and 23.

Surgical management of constipation

Surgery has also been used in the management of severe intractable constipation though this is usually reserved for the younger patients. Subtotal colectomy with ileorectal anastomosis has been the most popular operation performed though it is not universally successful. Kamm *et al.* (1989), in a study of 44 chronically constipated patients treated with colectomy, found that only 22 (50%) had normal bowel frequency post-operatively, 17 (39%) had diarrhoea with more than three stools passed per day with many experiencing faecal incontinence, and five (11%) had persistent constipation. Seventy-one percent of their patients still experienced abdominal pain post-operatively and ten patients needed treatment for psychiatric disorders though it is unclear whether this pre-dated the surgery.

Yoshioka and Keighley (1989), in their series of 40 patients, produced similar results and found that pre-operative anorectal studies did not assist in predicting surgical outcome. They recommended that surgery is contraindicated in people with psychiatric disease or major psychological problems.

Stabile *et al.* (1991) in a follow up to their groups earlier study (Kamm *et al.* 1989), compared the outcome of colectomy with ileorectal or caecorectal anastomosis for patients with idiopathic megarectum or megacolon (mean age 35 years). They found that 80% of these patients had normal bowel frequency post-operatively. None of the 11 patients who had an ileorectal anastomosis experienced recurrent constipation, unlike the 22 caecorectal anastomosis patients, three of whom required further surgery (conversion to ileorectal anastomosis) to correct recurrent constipation.

The demonstration of obstructed defaecation due to pelvic floor muscle contraction has lead to interest in pelvic floor surgery for these patients. Division of the puborectalis muscle has not been found to produce beneficial effects (Barnes *et al.*, 1985; Kamm *et al.*, 1988).

Anorectal myomectomy may help to alleviate pelvic floor outlet obstruction (Yoshioka and Keighley, 1987). Short term improvement has been reported in 60–70% of patients. The procedure involves the excision of a strip of the internal anal sphincter and rectal circular muscle over a length of 10–12cm. Full assessment of the procedure is awaited. Other surgical procedures have also been investigated but no satisfactory alternative has yet been found.

Spinal stimulators

There does appear to be some hope for spinal injured patients with severe constipation. MacDonagh *et al.* (1990) have assessed the effect of the implantation and use of an anterior sacral nerve root stimulator on bowel function in 12 consecutive spinal injured patients who had the stimulator implanted primarily as part of the management of their urinary voiding problems but who also had very severe problems with constipation necessitating regular manual evacuation or the use of reflex methods to empty their bowels.

These stimulators were initially developed to improve bladder emptying (Brindley, 1977). The stimulators are implanted intradurally to stimulate three pairs of nerve roots (S2, S3, S4) and connected to a receiver unit on the lower chest wall. Stimulation is applied by holding a transmitter over the implanted receiver and switching on a hand held unit.

Each individual pair of nerve roots could be stimulated separately or in combinations. A process of trial and error was used in an anorectal physiology laboratory to determine the optimum strength and intermittency of stimulation parameters to achieve the maximum recto-anal pressure gradient.

S2 stimulation tended to produce low pressure colorectal activity, S3 and to a lesser extent, S4 produced colorectal contraction. S4 stimulation produced the maximum anal pressure response. There was considerable inter-individual variation in the stimulation parameters which was also observed by Varma *et al.* (1986).

Continuous stimulation tended to produce rectal muscle fatigue which took five minutes or more to recover. This mode of stimulation did not successfully produce defaecation whereas intermittent stimulation produced defaecation in nine of the 12 patients in a simulated defaecation test. Six of these patients were subsequently able to defaecate using the stimulator alone.

In 11 of these patients the time taken to defaecate was shortened using the stimulator as well as being more frequent. The time spent in defaecation was significantly reduced and constipation was eradicated.

Implantation of the stimulator does require deafferentation of the sacral spinal cord and reflex defaecation using suppositories or anal digitisation was abolished. Patients unable to defaecate with the stimulator alone therefore had to perform manual evacuation of faeces once it reached the rectum but at least this allowed the rectum to be emptied in a predictable and manageable way.

References

Abd-el-Maeboud KH, El-Naggar T, El-Hawi EMM, Mahmoud SAR, Abd-el-Hay S. (1991) Rectal suppository: commonsense mode of insertion. *Lancet*; **338**: 798–800.

Andersson H, Bosaeus I, Falkheden T, Melkersson M. (1979) Transit time in constipated geriatric patients during treatment with a bulk laxative and bran: a comparison. *Scand J Gastroenterol*; **14**: 821–6.

Ardron ME, Main ANH. (1990) Management of constipation. *Br Med J*; **300**: 1400.

Barnes PRH, Hawley PR, Preston DM, Lennard-Jones JE. (1985) Experience of posterior division of the puborectalis muscle in the management of chronic constipation. *Br J Surg*; **72**: 475–7.

Bass P, Dennis S. (1981) The laxative effects of lactulose in normal and constipated subjects. *J Clin Gastroenterol*; 3 Suppl 1: **23**–8.

Binnie NR, Creasy G, Edmond P, Smith AN. (1988) The action of cisapride on the chronic constipation of paraplegia. *Paraplegia*; **26**: 151–8.

Brindley GS. (1977) An implant to empty the bladder and close the urethra. *J Neuro Neurosurg Psychiat*; **40**: 358–69.

Brocklehurst JC, Kirkland JL, Martin J, Ashford J. (1983) Constipation in long-stay elderly patients: its treatment and prevention by lactulose, poloxalkol-dihydroxyanthroquinolone and phosphate enemas. *Gerontol*; **29**: 181–4.

Brown JP. (1980) A review of the genetic effects of naturally occurring flavinoids, anthroquinolones and related compounds. *Mutation Res*; **75**: 243–77.

Burkitt DP, Walker ARP, Painter NS. (1972) Effect of dietary fibre on stools and transit-times, and its role in the causation of disease. *Lancet*; ii: 1408-11.

Clarke ANG, Scott JF. (1976) Wheat bran in dyschezia in the aged. *Age and Ageing*; **5**: 149–54.

Davis GR, Santa Ana CA, Morawski SG, Fordtran JS. (1980) Development of a lavage solution associated with minimal water and electrolyte absorption or secretion. *Gastroenterology*; **78**: 991–5.

Deiling DA, Fischer RA, Fernandez O. (1959) The therapeutic usefulness of Dulcalax. *Am J Dig Dis*; **4**: 311.

Donald IP, Smith RG, Cruikshank JG, Elton RA, Stoddart ME. (1985) A study of constipation in the elderly living at home. *Gerontology*; **31**: 112–18.

Edwards CA, Tomlin J, Read NW. (1988). Fibre and constipation. *Br J Clin*; **42**: 26–32.

Elazarion EJ, Shirachi DY, Jones JK. (1980) Educational approaches promoting optimal laxative use in long-term care patients. *J Chron Dis*; **33**: 613–26.

Foord KD, Morcos SK, Ward P. (1983) A comparison of Mannitol and Magnesium Citrate preparations for double-contrast barium enema. *Clin radiol*; **34**: 309–12.

Goodman J, Pang J, Bessman AN. (1976) Dioctyl sodium sulphosuccinate – an ineffective prophylactic laxative. *J Chron Dis*; **29**: 59–63.

Hamilton JW, Wagner J, Burdick BB, Bass P. (1988) Clinical evaluation of methylcellulose as a bulk laxative. *Dig Dis Sci*; **33**: 993–8.

Hardcastle JD, Mann CV. (1968) Study of large bowel peristalsis. **Gut**; **9**: 512–20.

Hardcastle JD, Wilkins JL. (1970) The action of sennosides and related compounds on human colon and rectum. *Gut*; **11**: 1038–42.

Harvard LRC, Hughes-Roberts HE. (1962) The treatment of constipation in mental hospitals. *Gut*; **3**: 85–90.

Julien JY, Barbeau A, Forgues D. (1983) Controle de l'utilasation des laxatifs dans un centre hospitalier de soins prolonges. *Union Medicale Du Canada*; **112**: 1054–6.

Kamm MA, Hawley PR, Lennard-Jones JE. (1988) Lateral division of the puborectalis muscle in the management of severe constipation. *Br J Surg*; **75**: 661–3.

Kamm MA, Hawley PR, Lennard-Jones JE. (1989) Outcome of colectomy for severe idiopathic constipation. *Gut*; **29**: 969–73.

Krevsky B, Malmud LS, Maurer AH, Somers MB, Siegel JA. (1987) The effect of oral cisapride on colonic transit. *Aliment Pharmacol Therapeut*; **1**: 239–304.

Lederer PC, Ellerman A, Schmidt H, Ernst V, Lux G. (1986) Effect of cisapride on sigmoid motility in healthy subjects and in diabetic enteropathy (DE) with constipation. *Digestion*; **37**: 110–13.

Loening-Baucke V. (1989) Factors determining outcome in children with chronic constipation and faecal soiling. *Gut*; **30**: 999–1006.

MacDonagh RP, Sun WM, Smallwood R, Forster D, Raed NW. (1990) Control of defaecation in patients with spinal injuries by stimulation of sacral anterior nerve roots. *Br Med J*; **300**: 1494–7.

MacLennan WJ, Pooler AFWM. (1975) A comparison of sodium picosulphate (Laxoberal) with standardised senna (Senokot) in geriatric patients. *Curr Med Res Opinion*; **2**: 641–7.

Madsen JL. (1990) Effects of cisapride on gastrointestinal transit in healthy humans. *Dig Dis Sci*; **35**: 1500–4.

Marcus SN, Heaton KW. (1986) Effects of a new concentrated wheat fibre preparation on intestinal transit, deoxycholic acid metabolism and composition of bile. *Gut*; **27**: 893–900.

Mori H, Sugie S, Niwa K, Takahshi M, Kawai K. (1985) Induction of intestinal tumours in rats by chrysazin. *Br J Cancer*; **52**: 781–3.

Mori H, Sugie S, Niwa K, Yoshimi W, Tanaka T, Hirono J. (1986) Carcinogenicity of chrysazin in large intestine and liver of mice. *Japan J Cancer Res* (Gann); **77**: 871–6.

Muller-Lissner SA. (1988) Effect of wheat bran on weight of stool and gastrointestinal transit time: a meta analysis. *Br Med J*; **296**: 615–17.

Muller-Lissner SA and the Bavarian Constipation Study Group. (1987) Treatment of chronic constipation with cisapride and placebo. *Gut*; **28**: 1033–8.

Nolan T, Debelle G, Oberteland F, Coffey C. (1991) Randomized trial of laxatives in the treatment of childhood encopresis. *Lancet*; **338**: 523–7.

Palmer KR, Khan AN. (1979) Oral mannitol: a simple and effective bowel preparation for barium enema. *Br Med J*; **2**: 1038.

Puxty JAH, Fox RA. (1986) Golytely: a new approach to faecal impaction in old age. *Age and Ageing*; **15**: 182–4.

Resende TL, (1989) Constipation, faecal incontinence, and the effects of exercise and abdominal massage on colonic activity in old age. *MSc thesis, University of Manchester*.

Smith I, Carr NM, Corrado O, Young A. (1987) Rectal necrosis after a phosphate enema. *Age and Ageing*; **16**: 328–30.

Smith RG, Currie JEJ, Walls ADF. (1978) Whole gut irrigation: a new treatment for constipation. *Br Med J*; **2**: 396–7.

Stabile G, Kamm MA, Hawley PR, Lennard-Jones JE. (1991) Colectomy for idiopathic megarectum and megacolon. *Gut*; **32**: 1538–40.

Sweeney JL, Hewett P, Riddel P, Hoffman DC. (1986) Rectal gangrene a compliaction of phosphate enema. *Med J Australia*; **144**: 374–5.

Tomlin J, Read NW. (1988) Laxative properties of indigestible plastic particles. *Br Med J*; **297**: 1175–6.

Twycross RG. (1989) Constipation in advanced cancer. *Geriat Med* (Supplement on Constipation); 19–22.

Varma JS, Binnie NR, Smith AN, Creasy G, Edmond P. (1986) Differential effects of sacral anterior root stimulation on anal sphincters and colorectal motility in spinally injured man. *Br J Surg*; **73**: 478–82.

Wesselius-DeCasparis A, Braadbaart S, Van den Bergh-Bohlken GE, Micica M. (1968) Treatment of chronic constipation with 'lactulose' syrup. Results of a double blind study. *Gut*; **9**: 84–6.

Yoshioka K, Keighley MRB. (1987) Randomised trial comparing anorectal myomectomy and controlled anal dilatation for outlet obstruction. *Br J Surg*; **74**: 1125–9.

Yoshioka K, Keighley MRB. (1989) Clinical results of colectomy for severe constipation. *Br J Surg*; **76**: 600–4.

19

Treatment of diarrhoea

The most important principle in the management of acute diarrhoea is to ensure adequate fluid and electrolyte replacement until the diarrhoea settles to avoid dehydration and metabolic abnormalities.

Acute or chronic diarrhoea in the elderly is often associated with faecal incontinence. In these patients use of antidiarrhoeal agents will help to alter stool consistency and restore continence to the majority whilst the cause is being sought and treated. If continence is not achieved quickly then application of a faecal collection device around the anus allows this to be achieved (see p. 170).

Traditionally codeine phosphate was the drug used in the treatment of diarrhoea. It prolongs gastrointestinal transit by stimulating opiate receptors to produce an increase in non-propulsive intestinal motility without increasing propulsive motility. Newer agents have been developed for the treatment of diarrhoea with interesting features that have been applied to the treatment of faecal incontinence or which may have applications in its treatment in the future.

Loperamide is a synthetic opiate which is devoid of opiate central nervous system side effects (Galambos et al., 1976). It has been shown to increase intestinal motility in man (Schiller et al., 1984; Kachel et al., 1986; Tytgat and Huibregtse, 1975). Fiaramonti et al. (1987) found that loperamide stimulated gastrointestinal motility in dogs when administered orally or subcutaneously but not with intracerebroventricular administration. The effect was blocked by intravenous administration of naloxone which indicates that the effect of loperamide is on peripheral opiate receptors. Naloxone has also been found to block the antidiarrhoeal action of loperamide (Piercey and Ruwart, 1979).

In a study of experimentally induced osmotic diarrhoea in pigs loperamide was shown to delay orocaecal transit whilst increasing small intestinal phase 3 migrating motor complex activity. This reduced the flow entering the colon where water absorption was increased by loperamide, thus reducing the diarrhoea (Theodorou *et al.*, 1991).

Loperamide has also been found to have an effect on the internal anal sphincter. Rattan and Culver (1987) performed their studies on anaesthetised opposums. They administered the muscle relaxant, pancuronium, to eliminate the effect of the external sphincter and found that loperamide given intra-arterially caused the internal sphincter pressure to increase. This effect was blocked by the prior administration of naloxone. This stimulatory effect was shortlived, lasting for between five and ten minutes and was not blocked by the neurotoxin tetrodoxin which suggests that the action of loperamide is directly on smooth muscle and is mediated by activation of opiate receptors.

Rattan and Culver (1987) also found that loperamide inhibited the normal relaxation of the internal sphincter that follows rectal distension for 1–3 hrs after an intra-arterial injection. It also blocked the usual inhibition of internal sphincter pressure that follows pre-sacral nerve stimulation. Salducci *et al.* (1982) have also shown that loperamide influences internal sphincter pressure and response to distension. They also demonstrated that alpha adrenoreceptor agonists can influence internal sphincter pressure.

In a clinical study Read *et al.* (1982) investigated the effects of loperamide 4mg tds on continence to a standard volume of rectally infused saline in 26 young and middle aged patients with faecal incontinence and chronic diarrhoea. Each patient also had anorectal manometry performed. Their double-blind cross-over trial compared treatment for one week with loperamide (4mg tds) with an identical placebo for one week. There was a significant reduction in incontinent episodes during the study and this was associated with a significant improvement in stool consistency and a reduction in stool weight during the loperamide period. Continence to rectally infused saline improved with a significant increase in the volume to first leak and an increase in the volume of saline retained during the test. Loperamide was also found to produce a slight but significant increase in anal resting pressure.

Similar studies have not been performed using codeine phosphate but it would appear that constipating drugs and in particular loperamide may prevent faecal incontinence by mechanisms other than by just changing stool consistency.

Other studies have provided other information about these drugs which can be used to guide treatment in the faecally incontinent patient.

O'Brien *et al.* (1988) found that loperamide is often ineffective when given in standard doses to patients with post vagotomy diarrhoea but high dose treatment (12–24mg/day) often produces a good response. They also found that some patients who failed to respond to loperamide responded well to codeine phosphate. Codeine phosphate was shown to delay intestinal transit more effectively if given at least one hour before meals as this allowed plasma levels to reach therapeutic levels. If given with meals both loperamide and codeine phospate will tend to pass through the small intestine before absorption can occur. The beneficial effects are therefore lost.

Loperamide has a long half life (15–40 hours) (Killinger *et al.*, 1979) and it may take several days before symptomatic improvement is seen.

Cholestyramine may help reduce diarrhoea in patients with bile salt malabsorption but at present it is unknown whether this is a significant factor in the production of diarrhoea in old age.

There are some other agents that are used in the treatment of severe diarrhoea which may have effects that are beneficial to patients with faecal incontinence. Fedorak and Field (1987) have reviewed the antidiarrhoeal effects of these drugs.

Clonidine, an alpha 2 adrenoceptor agonist (Jiang *et al.*, 1988), Somatostatin analogue (Moller *et al.*, 1988) and Odanesteron, a selective $5HT_3$ receptor antagonist (Talley *et al.*, 1990) have all been shown to slow intestinal transit.

Clonidine may be useful in patients with diarrhoea and autonomic neuropathy without inducing the usual central side effects, e.g. hypotension.

Subcutaneous treatment with somatostatin analogues is used in patients with rare hormonally mediated diarrhoea, e.g. VIPomas, and has also been used in AIDS patients with severe chronic diarrhoea but the lack of an oral preparation and the expense preclude its use at present in other patients with diarrhoea.

References

Fedorak RN, Field M. (1987) Antidiarrheal therapy. Prospects for new agents. *Dig Dis Sci*; **32**: 195–205.

Fioramonti J, Fargeas MJ, Bueno L. (1987) Stimulation of gastrointestinal motility by loperamide in dogs. *Dig Dis Sci*; **32**: 641–6.

Galambos JT, Hersh T, Schroder S, Wenger J. (1976) Loperamide: a new antidiarrheal agent in the treatment of chronic diarrhea. *Gastroenterology*; **70**: 1026–9.

Jiang Q, Sheldon RJ, Porreca F. (1988) Sites of clonidine action to inhibit gut propulsion in mice: demonstration of a central component. *Gastroenterology*; **95**: 1265–71.

Kachel G, Ruppin H, Hagel J, Barina W, Meinhardt M, Domschke W. (1986) Human intestinal motor activity and transport: Effects of a synthetic opiate. *Gastroenterology*; **90**: 85–93.

Killinger JM, Weintraub HS, Fuller BL. (1979) Human pharmacokinetics and comparative bioavailability of loperamide hydrochloride. *J Clin Pharmacol*; **19**: 211–8.

Moller N, Petrany G, Cassidy D, Sheldon WL, Johnston DG, Laker MF. (1988) Effects of the somatostatin analogue SMS 201-995 (sandostatin) on mouth-to-caecum transit time and absorption of fat and carbohydrates in normal man. *Clin Sci*; **75**: 345–50.

O'Brien JD, Thompson DG, McIntyre A, Burnham WR, Walker E. (1988) Effect of codeine and loperamide on upper intestinal transit and absorption in normal subjects and patients with postvagotomy diarrhoea. *Gut*; **29**: 312–318.

Piercey MF, Ruwart MJ. (1979) Naloxone blocks the antidiarrhoeal activity of loperamide. *Br J Pharmacol*; **66**: 373–375.

Rattan S, Culver PJ. (1987) Influence of loperamide on the internal anal sphincter in the oppossum. *Gastroenterology*; **93**: 121–8.

Read M, Read NW, Barber DC, Duthie HL. (1982) Effects of loperamide on anal sphincter function in patients complaining of chronic diarrhoea with faecal incontinence and urgency. *Dig Dis Sci*; **27**: 807–14.

Salducci J, Planche D, Naudy B. (1982) Physiological role of the internal anal sphincter and the external anal sphincter during micturition. In: Weinbeck M, (ed). *Motility of the Digestive Tract*; Raven Press, New York.

Schiller LR, Santa Ana CA, Morawski SG, Fordtran JS. (1984) Mechanism of the anti diarrheal effect of loperamide. *Gastroenterology*; **86**: 1475–80.

Talley NJ, Phillips SF, Haddad A, *et al.*, (1990) GR 38032F (Odanesteron), a selective 5HT$_3$ receptor antagonist, slows colonic transit in healthy man. *Dig Dis Sci*; **35**: 477–80.

Theodorou V, Fioramonti J, Hachet T, Bueno L. (1991) Absorptive and motor components of the antidiarrhoeal action of loperamide: an *in vivo* study in pigs. *Gut*; **32**: 1355–9.

Tytgat GN, Huibregtse K. (1975) Loperamide and ileostomy output – placebo controlled double-blind crossover study. *Lancet*; **ii**: 667.

20

Treatment of faecal incontinence secondary to cerebral disease

The main cause of faecal incontinence in patients with dementing illnesses is faecal loading. They tend to be unaware of the presence of faeces in the rectum and the need to defaecate. Treatment therefore should be aimed initially at alleviating this problem using the methods described in Chapter 19. Often the simple aim of ensuring that stool is firm in consistency, i.e. not too soft and not too hard, will restore continence. If these methods fail then it is generally accepted practice to implement a regimen of planned bowel evacuations.

Jarrett and Exton-Smith (1960) first described a regimen in which kaolin and morphine was given every morning to induce constipation and Senokot every evening to stimulate bowel evacuation the following morning.

There was little further research interest in this subject until Tobin and Brocklehurst (1986) performed their study of elderly residents in local authority residential homes. The vast majority of the incontinent residents in these homes had evidence of a dementing illness. The faecally incontinent patients were randomly allocated to either a treatment group or the control group. The active treatment group of patients who were faecally incontinent mainly due to their poor mental state were given codeine phosphate (30–60 mg/day) as the constipating drug with twice weekly enemas to induce defaecation. The faecally loaded patients had this treated with daily enemas until the bowel was clear, followed by regular laxatives.

There was a significant improvement in the treatment group with continence being restored to 60% of these patients compared to the 32% spontaneous improvement in the control group (see Table 5, p. 133). Thirty-six percent of their treatment group, however, were still incontinent at least once per week at the end of the study period. There was, however, a problem achieving compliance with the suggested treatment regimen. Only 13% of the patients who received the full treatment were still incontinent when reviewed after two months. Obtaining the full compliance of the patient and the medical and nursing staff is therefore very important when aiming to treat and prevent faecal incontinence in these patients. There also appears to be a trend in Tobin and Brocklehurst's (1986) results towards persistent incontinence in the patients who are incontinent because of their poor mental state as opposed to those who are incontinent primarily due to faecal loading.

Tobin and Brocklehurst's (1986) results are encouraging as they demonstrate that faecal incontinence can be 'cured'.

Rands and Malone Lee (1991) have also studied the management of faecal incontinence in patients with dementing illness. The setting for their study was in hospital long stay wards for the elderly mentally ill. Forty-six percent of their sample were chairbound. They studied patients on two wards within the same hospital. Patients on one ward which acted as a control ward were compared with a therapeutic trial group of patients. On the therapeutic trial ward constipated patients were given senna 7.5mg daily and micro-enemas twice weekly. Abdominal radiographs were performed to identify the degree of colonic faecal loading and all patients were given a high fibre diet. On the control ward no intervention took place apart from a recording of bowel habit.

Compliance rates with the suggested treatment in the therapeutic trial group were 54% for senna and 46% for the micro-enemas. During the eight week study period there was no change in the rate of urinary or faecal incontinence on the treatment ward but faecal incontinence was found to be worse on the control ward at the end of this time. There was no change in the extent of constipation identified using the abdominal radiographs on the treatment ward. Faecal loading assessed by digital rectal examination was found to be reduced in the treatment group.

Interpretation of the results of these two studies (Tobin and Brocklehurst, 1986; Rands and Malone-Lee, 1991) is not easy as firstly they did not study the same type of patients. One would expect patients in long stay wards for the elderly mentally ill to have more mental and physical problems than their counterparts in local authority residential homes.

Both studies had treatment regimens that could be criticised. Rands and Malone-Lee (1991) did not take account of stool consistency when planning patients' treatment and routinely administered a high fibre diet despite the evidence that most elderly patients with faecal loading are loaded with very soft faeces (Barrett, 1988) which is more likely to leak than firm faeces (Barrett *et al.*, 1990) and that an increase in fibre intake tends to increase the rate of faecal incontinence (Ardron and Main, 1990). The lack of benefit may be due to the use of fibre negating the beneficial effects of the treatment given. The poor compliance rates also make interpretation difficult.

Tobin and Brocklehurst (1986) out of necessity used a fixed regimen with constipating drug plus twice weekly microenemas in their study. In clinical practice, however, the constipating drug is not always required.

The regimen of planned defaecation ideally therefore should comprise an enema or suppository 1–3 times per week, though this is usually twice weekly with a constipating drug (loperamide or codeine phosphate) being given to patients who have a tendency to faecal leakage between these enemas.

The two studies demonstrate the difficulties that are encountered when trying to obtain compliance with the treatment regimens. Staff attitudes about the 'inevitable' faecal incontinence are one barrier to overcome but even more difficult to overcome is patient resistance to the treatment. Many patients on long stay wards for the elderly mentally ill exhibit severe behavioural difficulties which prevent the administration of medication especially if this is to be given rectally as an enema.

These two factors probably account for the continuing high prevalence of faecal incontinence in continuing care homes and hospital long stay wards. It is hoped that staff education will in the long term lead to changes in management protocols in these settings and a reduction in the prevalence of faecal incontinence.

The bigger challenge, however, is the group of patients with severe behavioural problems which render the management of their incontinence (or more accurately, inappropriate defaecation) difficult if not impossible using current methods which tend to depend upon the introduction of rectal preparations. These patients have a tendency to be soiled numerous times per day every day and often have other abnormal behavioural traits which include faecal smearing (personal observations).

Some success in continence control can be achieved in these patients by administering a potent laxative orally once weekly to produce a predictable bowel clearance on a single day to replace the continuous faecal leakage that often occurs in these patients (personal observations). Picolax can usually be relied upon to clear the bowel hence its use in bowel preparation for barium enema (Foord *et al.*, 1983). It is however difficult for frail elderly patients to control this and impossible for the elderly confused patient to do so. Patients therefore should be carefully supervised on 'Picolax day' as they are prone to severe faecal incontinence in the 24 hours after its administration. This can be minimised by using very small doses of Picolax (e.g. ½ sachet as a single dose).

For patients with stool which is soft in consistency sodium picosulphate alone is the preferred agent as continence is less likely to be compromised if the potent osmotic action of magnesium citrate can be avoided. Once massive faecal loading has been cleared, a once weekly treatment is usually sufficient for these patients typically as they have slow transit constipation with whole gut transit times in excess of 14 days (Brocklehurst and Khan, 1969). They therefore tend to accumulate sufficient faeces over a seven day period for a further bowel clearance to be required to prevent the occurrence of faecal soiling during everyday activities.

Another potential way of minimising faecal leakage on 'Picolax day' is to use a faecal collecting bag but unfortunately patients with severe dementing illnesses tend to pull the bag off. There is scope therefore for further improvement in the management of these patients whose problems may prove to be intractable.

References

Ardron ME, Main ANH. (1990) Management of constipation. *Br Med J*; **300**: 1400.

Barrett JA. (1988) Effect of wheat bran on stool size. *Br Med J*; **296**: 1127–8.

Barrett JA, Brocklehurst JC, Kiff ES, Ferguson G, Faragher EB. (1990) Rectal motility studies in geriatric patients with faecal incontinence. *Age and Ageing*; **19**: 311–17.

Brocklehurst JC, Khan MY. (1969) A study of faecal stasis in old age and the use of 'Dorbanex' in its prevention. *Gerontol Clin*; **11**: 293–300.

Foord KD, Morcos SK, Ward P. (1983) A comparison of Mannitol and Magnesium Citrate preparations for double-contrast barium enema. *Clin radiol*; **34**: 309–12.

Jarrett AS, Exton-Smith AN. (1960) Treatment of faecal incontinence. *Lancet*; **i**: 925.

Rands G, Malone-Lee J. (1991) Urinary and faecal incontinence in long stay wards for the elderly mentally ill; prevalence and difficulties in management. *Health Trends*; **22**: 161–3.

Tobin GW, Brocklehurst JC. (1986) Faecal incontinence in residential homes for the elderly: prevalence, aetiology and management. *Age and Ageing*; **15**: 41–6.

21

Treatment of anorectal incontinence

The principles for treating patients with anorectal incontinence are similar to those described in Chapters 18 and 19. The majority of patients are able to regain continence by adjusting the consistency of their faeces so that it is firm, as hard faeces tends to be difficult to defaecate and soft or liquid faeces tends to be difficult to control with consequent involuntary leakage. There are some patients who, despite modification of their stool consistency and defaecation habits, continue to experience faecal incontinence. There are other treatment options which may help. These include biofeedback, electrical stimulation and surgery.

These treatments are mainly aimed at young and middle aged incontinent patients who are incontinent due to the presence of an isolated anorectal abnormality. Some elderly people may also benefit from this approach.

Biofeedback

A number of biofeedback techniques have been assessed in the management of anorectal incontinence. Some studies have produced good results with success rates of up to 70% (Cerulli et al., 1979, Macleod, 1987; Wald and Tunuguntla, 1984; Miner et al., 1990) including a study of elderly patients who were incontinent of solid stool (Whitehead et al., 1985). Loening Baucke (1990), however, did not find any significant improvement with biofeedback.

Miner et al. (1990) studied 25 incontinent patients aged 17–76 and divided them into an active biofeedback retraining group and a sham retraining group who had the same procedures performed but did not receive any instruction. Seventy six percent of the biofeedback patients had a reduction of at least 75% in the frequency of their incontinent episodes at the end of the biofeedback retraining. Fifty percent had no incontinent episodes at all. At the two year follow up three of the original 25 had proceeded to surgical treatment and another three were lost to follow up. Seventeen of the remaining 19 originally improved and this was sustained. The other two reported having a better quality of life as they had more time to reach the toilet and were able to go out of the house again after the retraining although they had no reduction in the number of incontinent episodes.

Miner *et al.*'s (1990) method involved two phases over a two month period with a mixture of formal sessions utilising rectal balloon distension and measurement of anal pressure to provide feedback to the patient. Phase I was a period of sensory retraining and was followed in phase II by training sessions to improve external sphincter strength and sessions of coordination training. Miner *et al.*'s training method is described in detail in the original paper.

Miner *et al.* (1990) also evaluated some of the factors which have been thought to be responsible for the success of biofeedback retraining. They confirmed Loening Baucke's (1990) finding that biofeedback does not lead to any change in anal resting or squeeze pressures. The main changes that occur are a reduction in the threshold volume for the sensation of rectal distension and the correction of sensory delays. It is not surprising therefore that the significant improvements in both continence and sensory awareness occurred during the sensory retraining in phase I with some further improvement in continence in phase II.

Improved sensation may allow longer warning from the entry of stool into the rectum to defaecation, enhanced perception of small stool and awareness of stool before reflex internal sphincter relaxation occurs.

Patients in the sham training groups also had a significant though modest reduction in sensory threshold. Psychological factors, e.g. reduced anxiety, may account for this and for the spontaneous improvement in continence that occurred in 50% of this group. Continence during saline infusion tests was not affected by biofeedback training which suggests that incontinence to liquid stool may persist in these patients and perhaps explains Loening Baucke's (1990) results as all the treatment patients in that study were incontinent of liquid stool.

Psychological aspects of biofeedback will be discussed in more detail in Chapter 23. Sensory retraining does appear to offer a safe inexpensive method of treatment for anorectal incontinence that should be considered if conventional conservative treatment has not been successful. There is also some preliminary data suggesting beneficial effects with a biofeedback regimen in the management of constipated patients with obstructed defaecation (Kawimbe *et al.*, 1991).

Electrical stimulation

Pelvic floor muscle re-education has been included as part of the management of urinary stress incontinence for a long time. There is however no established practice in the use of similar regimens in the treatment of anorectal incontinence.

The effect of electrical stimulation upon striated muscle is the subject of increasing research interest at present and this research is likely to lead soon to the introduction of alternative protocols for muscle stimulation.

Chronic electrical stimulation given for several hours daily over weeks or months has been shown to produce adaptations of innervated muscle (Pette 1986). The contractile properties of skeletal muscle depend upon the impulse activity imposed upon it by the motor neurone (Buller *et al.*, 1960, Vbrova, 1963; Salmons and Vbrova, 1969) and the histochemical profile reflects the normal use of the muscle (Pette and Vbrova, 1985; Kugelberg *et al.*, 1968). Transformation of one type of muscle fibre to another can be achieved by controlling the input to the muscle (Nemeth, 1982). Chronic electrical stimulation increases the blood supply and decreases fatiguability of mammalian muscle (Hudlicka *et al.*, 1977) and human muscle (Scott *et al.*, 1984, 1985).

The earliest methods of electrical stimulation in clinical practice used faradic stimulation with a frequency of 50Hz. This stimulation however may be potentially harmful as Kernell *et al.* (1987) have shown that high frequency stimulation of skeletal muscle often results in a decrease of maximum tetanic force. Force does appear to be maintained with mixed frequency stimulation programmes (Rutherford and Jones, 1988; Oldham and Stanley, 1989). This principle was successfully used by Faragher *et al.* (1987) in the re-education of the facial muscles using eutrophic stimulation in patients with Bell's palsy.

Conventional physiotherapy techniques have not been very successful in the management of the pelvic floor muscle weakness in patients with anorectal incontinence. This may be because pelvic floor muscle exercises are dependent upon intact sensory and motor pathways.

Electrical stimulation for stress urinary incontinence using faradism (Scott *et al.*, 1969) or interferential therapy (McQuire, 1975) have produced very variable results as have the comparative studies of electrotherapy and exercises (Wilson *et al.*, 1987). Moderate degrees of success have been achieved in the treatment of the less severe cases of stress urinary incontinence (Kegal, 1948; Jones, 1950; Stoddard, 1983; Plevnik, 1985; Laycock 1987; Peattie *et al.*, 1988) while patients with anorectal incontinence have shown no improvement with faradism and pelvic floor exercises (Parks, 1975) or with interferential therapy (Sylvester and Keilty, 1987). Some studies report favourable results from electrical stimulation of the pelvic floor muscles (Matheson and Keighley, 1981; Caldwell, 1963; Hopkinson and Lightwood, 1966) but this has not been reproduced elsewhere (Collins *et al.*, 1969).

Faragher *et al.*'s (1987) good results with Bell's palsy patients lead Mills *et al.* (1990) to perform eutrophic stimulation on the muscles of the pelvic floor. A preponderance of type 1 muscle fibres, similar to the facial muscles, has been found in the sphincter muscles (Gosling, 1979; Gosling *et al.*, 1981; Gilpin *et al.*, 1989) which lead Mills *et al.* to believe that they may be able to decrease sphincter muscle fatiguability by electrical stimulation.

Mills *et al.* studied 36 incontinent patients in a pilot study on the use of an eutrophic electrical stimulator on the pelvic floor muscles. They had all been incontinent for at least three years. Ninety percent of them had undergone at least one pelvic operation, 63% two or more and 36% three or more. Sixteen stopped the treatment before the end of the programme due to either anal pain, family commitments or lack of response.

The stimulation was delivered between an electrode placed over the sacrum and another electrode placed over the anus. Patients were instructed in how to position the electrodes and operate the portable battery powered stimulator during the initial treatment session with the physiotherapist following which they self-administered the treatment with telephone help when required. The initial settings on the stimulator were set for 10 minutes treatment at 10Hz frequency using pulse widths between 80 microseconds and 200 microseconds at a rate of four seconds on, four seconds off. The treatment was then increased over the next few days to 60 minutes/day. The frequency was increased in patients who did not respond to 20Hz, 27Hz or 33Hz. The treatment lasted for 12 weeks.

Twenty of their patients completed the treatment programme. Thirteen (65%) of these improved or were much improved. Six of these patients regained continence but in five of these this regressed when the treatment was stopped. One of these patients, on entry to the study, was waiting to have a colostomy performed following a failed postanal repair. Continence was regained in this patient by restarting the treatment three times weekly. Mills *et al.* (1990) suggested that a good result was more likely when the weakness was limited to the external anal sphincter. Patients with combined internal and external anal sphincter weakness appeared less likely to benefit.

In the Mills *et al.* (1990) study, the patients all clearly had very severe problems. Results are awaited from their follow up study of patients with external anal sphincter weakness treated with eletrical stimulation before proceeding to surgery rather than on failed surgical patients.

Binnie *et al.* (1990) have reported on the use of an electrical stimulator which delivered 10Hz square wave 0·1ms stimuli via electrodes applied in the midline at the base of the clitoris. The mean stimulation voltage was 135 volts. The stimulator produced a significant immediate rise in external sphincter EMG activity and in anal resting pressure. Self-administered treatment was given for five minutes three times daily for eight weeks. At the end of this period seven of their eight incontinent patients had regained continence to both solids and liquids. A significant rise was found in anal resting pressure and squeeze pressure. The external anal sphincter pressure elicited by coughing was also found to be higher after the course of electrical stimulation.

Sackier and Woods (1989) have also reported encouraging results from their pilot study using a peranal electrode which makes contact with the anal mucosa at the anorectal angle and in the middle of the canal. They started treatment by admitting patients to hospital for five days. The stimulation given was 35 Hz with a pulse width 200 microseconds with a contraction time of four seconds and relaxation time of six seconds. The stimulation voltage was in the range 0–6 volts. The treatment was given 5 min/hr, 12 times in the first five days then patients were asked to use the device at home for 15 mins four times during the day and also overnight. Seventeen of their patients with faecal incontinence regained continence after 6 weeks' treatment. None of their patients withdrew or complained of discomfort from the treatment. Two of their patients regressed when treatment ceased but improved again when it was restarted.

These pilot studies suggest that in the future there will be a role for electrical stimulation in the management of anorectal incontinence but at present it is limited to being a research treatment until it has been developed further as there is currently no agreement on how it should be performed.

One of the main requirements for this treatment is for the machinery and electrodes to be portable, easy to operate and to reliably deliver the stimulation. Studies of patients with urinary incontinence treated at home have demonstrated that anal (Plevnik *et al.*, 1986; Eriksen *et al.*, 1987) or vaginal (Fall, 1984) electrodes are effective at delivering the stimulus.

Eriksen and Eik-nes (1989) reported 72% success rates for electrostimulation given for at least three months in the management of stress urinary incontinence. Twenty percent of their original patients, however, had to drop out because of anal pain and discomfort.

Surgical treatment

Anorectal incontinence may occur due to either injury of the external anal spincter or its nerve supply both of which may occur during childbirth and may co-exist (Snooks *et al.*, 1985).

Obstetric tears of the external anal sphincter have been managed by surgical repair of the tear. Laurberg *et al.* (1988) found that approximately 50% of women with these tears also had evidence of pudendal nerve damage and that the results of the surgical repair whilst excellent in patients without evidence of nerve damage were disappointing in those with nerve damage. Further surgery, e.g. postanal repair, may restore continence in these patients.

The main indication for surgery is anorectal incontinence that has not responded to conservative measures. Keighley (1987) comments that approximately 25% of patients presenting to his surgical practice respond well to conservative measures. He also comments that age is not a contraindication to surgery and that excellent results with complete restoration of continence have been obtained in patients aged over 70 years. Faecal incontinence in elderly people with disabilities is usually due to a combination of factors and the proportion of elderly incontinent patients who have pure anorectal incontinence is small and accounts for less than 5% of these patients.

The operation of postanal repair was first performed by Parks in 1961 with the aim of recreating the anorectal angle (Parks, 1967) (Fig. 35). The surgical technique has been reviewed by Keighley (1987). The main part of the procedure is to suture the two limbs of the puborectalis muscle together to recreate the puborectalis sling. The anorectal angle has been shown, however, not to be relevant to the outcome of surgery as a number of studies have failed to show any correlation between the angle and outcome and have failed to show any change in the angle after surgery (Miller *et al.*, 1988, Miller *et al.*, 1989, Womack *et al.*, 1988).

Henry and Simson (1985) reviewed the results of all the postanal repair operations performed for anorectal incontinence at St Marks Hospital, London between 1978 and 1983. Two hundred and forty-two patients were operated upon with 583% of the total having continence restored or considerably improved which included 69% of the patients aged between 50 and 69 years. The results, however, were disappointing in patients aged over 69 years with only 50% achieving continence.

In other studies approximately 90% of the middle aged patients had improved when reviewed at least 12 months post-operatively of whom 30–40% had completely regained continence (Miller *et al.*, 1988, Womack *et al.*, 1988, Keighley and Fielding, 1983, Yoshioka *et al.*, 1987).

Studies of the effects of postanal repair have produced inconsistent results possibly due to the small number of patients in the samples and slight variations in surgical technique between centres. Miller *et al.* (1989) suggest that patients with a successful outcome have a significant increase in anal squeeze pressure postoperatively but Womack *et al.* (1988) did not find any change in squeeze pressure or resting pressure. Miller *et al.* (1989), however, demonstrated significant improvement in upper anal canal sensation assessed by mucosal electrosensitivity

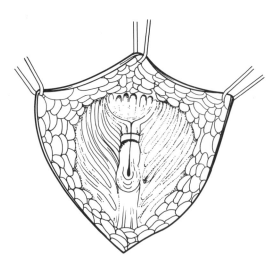

Fig. 35 Diagrammatic representation of the midline plication of the puborectalis muscles which is performed during the operation of postanal repair

postoperatively which they suggest may be due to lax anal mucosa being drawn back up into the anal canal.

Yoshioka *et al.* (1988) suggested that low anal resting and squeeze pressures, abnormal pelvic floor and perineal descent and a short anal canal were predictive factors of a poor outcome after postanal repair. Scott *et al.* (1990), however, did not find any evidence of very low anal resting pressure predicting poor outcome after postanal repair in a study of 62 patients.

Laurberg *et al.* (1990) studied 18 patients 9–35 months after they had a postanal repair for anorectal incontinence. None had evidence of pudendal neuropathy pre-operatively. Seventy two percent of their group had a good result with surgery. They were unable to identify any consistent change in anal pressures but found a significant increase in pudendal terminal motor latency even in patients who had a good result. They suggest that postanal repair may accelerate neurogenic damage to the pelvic floor muscles either from trauma to the innervation of the pelvic floor muscles during the operative dissection or by the entrapment of the pudendal nerves in fibrous tissue.

Keighley (1987) suggested that the results of postanal repair in patients who have previously had a rectopexy for rectal prolapse are disappointing. Faecal incontinence complicates rectal prolapse in 70–80% of patients and is most common in elderly women. Abdominal rectopexy was considered the operation of choice for rectal prolapse. Keighley *et al.*, (1983) reported achieving complete control of the prolapse postoperatively in 173 of their series of 176 patients most of whom were elderly. Twenty one of the operations were performed under local anaesthetic. Sixty percent of their patients who were incontinent pre-operatively had their continence restored but clearly many continued

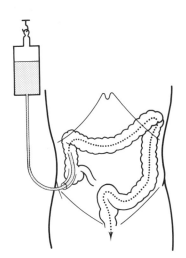

Fig. 36 Diagrammatic representation of a system which enables antegrade continence enemas to be administered through a non-refluxing catheterisable appendicocaecostomy in the management of intractable faecal incontinence

to experience faecal incontinence and needed to wear some form of protection. Difficulty with rectal evacuation is also experienced by at least 60% of patients after rectopexy though some of these patients had to strain or were constipated pre-operatively.

Alternatives treatments including encircling perianal suture of 'Teflon' wire and other perineal approaches have been discussed in a recent editorial (Anonymous, 1991). The results tend to be poor with a high frequency of recurrent rectal prolapse.

There is clearly a need for larger prospective studies to further evaluate and develop the surgical treatment of anorectal incontinence and their long term effects. Rectal surgeons are beginning to evaluate the implantation of artificial sphincter devices similar to those used by urologists in the management of some patients with severe urinary incontinence (Anonymous, 1989). The few small studies performed have been discussed in detail by Snooks (1992).

Malone *et al.*, (1990) have also reported the use of antegrade enemas administered via a non-refluxing appendicocaecostomy (Fig. 36) in the management of intractable faecal incontinence in five patients who were due to have colostomy performed as a last resort in the management of their severe faecal incontinence. They found that giving an antegrade enema via the stoma for 30 minutes on alternate days whilst the patient is sitting on a toilet produces a satisfactory bowel clearance and prevented faecal leakage in their patients during the interval between enemas. Prolonged follow up has not been possible so far but the early results are very encouraging with all the early patients regaining control of the evacuation of their bowels. Faecal leakage through the stoma is avoided by using the same technique to create the appendicocaecostomy that is employed in fashioning continent stomas in the surgical management of urinary incontinence.

References

Anonymous. (1989) Neurobiology of incontinence. *Lancet*; **ii**: 1078–9.

Anonymous. (1991) Rectal prolapse. *Lancet*; **338**: 605–6.

Binnie NR, Kawimbe BM, Papachrysostomou M, Smith AN. (1990) Use of the pudendo-anal reflex in the treatment of neurogenic faecal incontinence. *Gut*; **31**: 1051–5.

Buller AJ, Eccles JC, Eccles RM. (1960) Interactions between motor neurones and muscles in respect of the characteristic speeds of their responses. *J Physiology*. 150: 399–419.

Caldwell KPS. (1963) The electrical control of sphincter incompetence. *Lancet*; **ii**: 174–5.

Cerulli MA, Nikoomanesh P, Schuster MM. (1979) Progress in biofeedback conditioning for faecal incontinence. *Gastroenterology*; **76**: 742–6.

Collins CD, Brown BH, Duthie HL. (1969) An assessment of intraluminal electrical stimulation for anal incontinence. *Br J Surg*; **56**: 542–6.

Eriksen BC, Bergmann S, Mjolnerod OK. (1987) Effect of anal electrostimulation with the 'Incontan' device in women with urinary incontinence. *Br J Obstet Gynaecol*; **94**: 147–156.

Eriksen BC, Eik-nes SH. (1989) Long-tern electrostimulation of the pelvic floor: primary therapy in female stress incontinence? *Urol Int*; **44**: 90–5.

Fall M. (1984) Does electrostimulation cure urinary incontinence. *J Urol*; **131**: 664–7.

Faragher D, Kidd GL, Tallis R. (1987) Eutrophic stimulation for Bell's Palsy. *Clin Rehab*; **1**: 265–271.

Gilpin SA, Gosling JA, Smith ARB, Warrell D. (1989) The pathogenesis of genito-urinary prolapse and stress incontinence of urine. A histological and histochemical study. *Br J Obstet Gynaecol*; **96**: 15–23.

Gosling JA. (1979) The structure of the bladder and urethra in relation to function. *Urol Cli N America*; **6**: 31–8.

Gosling JA, Dixon JS, Critchley HOD, Thompson SA. (1981) A comparative study of the human external anal sphincter and periurethral levator ani muscle. *Br J Urol*; **53**: 35–41.

Henry MM, Simson JNL. (1985) Results of postanal repair: a retrospective study. *Br J Surg*; **72**(Suppl); S17–S19.

Hopkinson BR, Lightwood R. (1966) Electrical treatment of anal incontinence. *Lancet*; **i**: 297–8.

Hudlicka O, Brown M, Cotter M, Smith M, Vrbova G. (1977) The effect of long term stimulation of fast muscles on their bloodflow, metabolism and ability to withstand fatigue. *Pflugers Archiv Eur J Physiol*; **169**: 141–9.

Jones E. (1950) The role of active exercise in pelvic muscle physiology. *Western J surg*; **58**: 1–10.

Kawimbe BM, Papachrysostomou M, Binnie NR, Clare N, Smith AN. (1991) Outlet obstruction constipation (anismus) managed by biofeedback. *Gut*; **32**: 1175–9.

Kegal AH. (1948) Prolonged resistance exercises in the functional restoration of the perineal muscles. *Am J Obstet Gynecol*; **56**: 238–48.

Keighley MRB, Fielding JWL, Alexander-Williams J. (1983) Results of Marlex mesh abdominal rectopexy for rectal prolapse in 100 consecutive patients. *Br J Surg*; **70**: 229–32.

Keighley MRB, Fielding JWL. (1983) Management of faecal incontinence and results of surgical treatment. *Br J Surg*; **70**: 463–8.

Keighley MRB. (1987) How I do it. Postanal repair. *Int J Colorect Dis*; **2**: 236–9.

Kernell D, Eerbeek O, Vrhey BA, Donselaar D. (1987) Effects of physiological amounts of high and low rate chronic stimulation on fast twitch muscle of the cat hind limb. I. Speed and force related properties. *J Neurophysiol*; **58**: 598–613.

Kugelberg E, Edstrom L. (1968). Differential histochemical effects of muscle contraction on phosphorylase and glycogen in various types of muscle fibres. *J Neurol Neurosurg Psychiat*; **31**: 415–23.

Laurberg S, Swash M, Henry MM. (1988) Delayed external sphincter repair for obstetric tear. *Br J Surg*; **75**: 786–8.

Laurberg S, Swash M, Henry MM. (1990) Effect of postanal repair on progress of neurogenic damage to the pelvic floor. *Br J Surg*; **77**: 519–22.

Laycock J. (1987) Graded exercises for the pelvic floor muscles in the treatment of urinary incontinence. *Physio*; **73**: 371–3.

Loening-Baucke V. (1990) Efficacy of biofeedback training in improving faecal incontinence and anorectal physiologic function. *Gut*; **31**: 1395–1402.

Macleod JH. (1987) Management of anal incontinence by biofeedback. *Gastroenterology*; **93**: 291–4.

Malone PS, Ransley PG, Kiely EM. (1990) Preliminary report: the antegrade continence enema. *Lancet*; **336**: 1217–18.

Matheson DM, Keighley MRB. (1981) Manometric evaluation of rectal prolapse and faecal incontinence. *Gut*; **22**: 126–9.

McQuire WA. (1975) Electrotherapy and exercises for stress incontinence and urinary frequency. *Physiotherapy*; **61**: 305–7.

Miller R, Bartolo DCC, Locke-Edmunds JC, Mortensen NJMcC. (1988) Prospective study of conservative treatment and operative treatment for faecal incontinence. *Br J Surg;* **75**: 101–5.

Miller R, Orrom WJ, Cornes H, Duthie G, Bartolo DCC. (1989) Anterior sphincter plication and levatorplasty in the treatment of faecal incontinence. *Br J Surg;* **76**: 1058–60.

Mills PM, Deakin M, Kiff ES. (1990) Percutaneous electrical stimulation for ano-rectal incontinence. *Physiotherapy;* **76**: 433–8.

Miner PB, Donnelly TC, Read NW. (1990) Investigation of mode of action of biofeedback in treatment of faecal incontinence. *Dig Dis Sci;* **35**: 1291–98.

Nemeth PM. (1982) Electrical stimulation of denervated muscle prevents decreases in oxidative enzymes. *Muscle and Nerve;* February: 134–9.

Oldham JA, Stanley JE. (1989) Rehabilitation of atrophied muscle in the rheumatoid arthritic hand: a comparison of two methods of electrical stimulation. *Br J Hand Surg;* **14**: 294–7.

Parks AG. (1967) Post-anal perineorrhaphy for rectal prolapse. *Proc Roy Soc Med;* **60**: 920–1.

Parks AG. (1975) Ano-rectal incontinence. *Proc Roy Soc Med;* **59**: 477–82.

Peattie AB, Plevnik S, Stanton SL. (1988) Vaginal cones: A conservative method of treating genuine stress incontinence. *Br J Obstet Gynaecol;* **95**: 1049–53.

Pette D. (1986) Skeletal muscle adaptatio in response to chronic stimulation. In: Nix WA., Vrbova G. (eds). *Electrical Stimulation and Neuromuscular Disorders.* Springer-Verlag, Berlin.

Pette D, Vbrova G. (1985) Neural control of phenotype expression in mammalian muscle fibre. *Muscle and Nerve;* **8**: 676–89.

Plevnik S. (1985) A new method for testing and strengthening pelvic floor muscles. Proceedings of the 15th Annual General Meeting, International Continence Society, London.

Plevnik S, Janez J, Vrtacnik P, Trsinar B, Vodusek DB. (1986) Short-term electrical stimulation: home treatment for urinary incontinence. *World J Urol;* **4**: 24–6.

Rutherford OM, Jones DA. (1988) Contractile properties and fatiguability of the human adductor pollicis and first dorsal interosseus: a comparison of the effects of two chronic stimulation patterns. *J Neurol Sci;* **85**: 319–31.

Sackier JM, Woods CB. (1989) The anal sphincter. In: Rose FC, Jones R, Vbrova G. Neuromuscular Stimulation. Basic concepts and clinical implications. *Comprehensive Neuro Rehab;* **3**: 331–50.

Salmons S, Vbrova G. (1969) The influence of activity on some contractile characteristics of mammalian fast and slow muscles. J Physiol; **201**: 535–49.

Scott ADN, Henry MM, Phillips RKS. (1990) Clinical assessment and anorectal manometry before postanal repair: failure to predict outcome. *Br J Surg;* **77**: 628–9.

Scott BO, Green VM, Couldrey BM. (1969) Pelvic faradism: investigation of methods. *Physiotherapy;* **55**: 302.

Scott OM, Vrbova G, Dubowitz V. (1984) Effect of nerve stimulation on normal and diseased human muscle in Serratrice, G (ed) *Neuromuscular Disease;* Raven Press, New York.

Scott OM, Vrbova G, Hude SA, Dubowitz V. (1985) Effects of chronic low frequency electrical stimulation on normal human tibialis anterior muscle. *J Neurol Neurosurg Psychiat;* **48**: 774–81.

Snooks SJ. (1992) Faecal incontinence. Treatment: looking ahead to the role of prostheses. In: Henry MH, Swash M (eds). *Coloproctology and the Pelvic Floor;* pp. 287–9. Butterworth-Heinemann, Oxford.

Snooks SJ, Henry MM, Swash M. (1985) Faecal incontinence due to external anal sphincter division in childbirth is associated with damage to the innervation of the pelvic floor musculature: a double pathology. *Br J Obstet Gynaecol*; **92**: 824–8.

Stoddard GD. (1983) Research project into the effects of pelvic floor exercises in genuine stress incontinence. *Physiotherapy*; **69**: 148–9.

Sylvester KL, Keilty SE. (1987). A pilot study to investigate the use of interferential therapy in the treatment of anorectal incontinence. *Physiotherapy*; **73**: 207–8.

Vbrova G. (1963) The effect of motor neurone activity on the speed of contraction of striated muscle. *J Physiol*; **169**: 513–26.

Wald A, Tunuguntla AK. (1984) Anorectal sensorimotor dysfunction in faecal incontinence and diabetes mellitus. Modification with biofeedback therapy. *New Eng J Med. 310: 1282–7.*

*Whitehead WE, Burgio KL, Engel BT. (1985) Biofeedback treatment of faecal incontinence in geriatric patients. J Amer Geriat Soc; **33**: 320–4.*

Wilson PD, Al Samarrai T, Deakin M, Kolbe E, Brown ADG. (1987) The objective assessment of physiotherapy for female genuine stress incontinence. *Br J Obstet Gynaec*; **94**: 575–82.

Womack NR, Morrison JFB, Williams NS. (1988) Prospective study of the effects of postanal repair in neurogenic faecal incontinence. *Br J Surg*; **75**: 48–52.

Yoshioka K, Hyland G, Keighley MRB. (1987) Clinical and physiological evaluation of postanal repair. *Gut*; **28**: A1362.

Yoshioka K, Hyland G, Keighley MRB. (1988) Physiological changes after postanal repair and parameters predicting recovery. Br J Surg; **75**: 1220–4

22

Treatment of intractable faecal incontinence

Tobin and Brocklehurst's (1986) study of the treatment of faecal incontinence in the elderly suggests that most of these patients should regain full control over the emptying of their bowels if the methods described in Chapters 18–21 are followed.

Unfortunately some of these patients have persistent faecal incontinence despite these measures. The management of these patients depends upon their general health and overall well-being. Younger patients may be considered for surgery but this does not always correct the problem (see p. 161) as many remain incontinent of both urine and faeces despite anorectal surgery. Colostomy may be considered as a last resort in these patients when all other treatment options have been exhausted. Surgical treatment is rarely indicated in the frail elderly.

The management of elderly patients with intractable faecal incontinence is mainly based upon containment of faecal leakage using one of the small range of products that are available. The main products used for this purpose are the disposable incontinence pads. These comprise an absorbent pulp enclosed within a coverstock. The surface of the pad next to the perineum is permeable as the main use of these pads is to contain urinary incontinence. The cover on the outer surface is non-permeable. A variety of shapes and sizes are available to suit different patients' needs. Faecally incontinent patients usually require either a diaper or large shaped pads which are normally kept in position using stretch net elastic pants or a diaper (Fig. 37).

Containment of faecal incontinence using this method does not avoid faecal soiling of the skin or prevent the smell that surrounds the incontinent patient who has had 'an accident'. It is difficult to maintain personal hygiene and dignity with these products. Every effort should therefore be made by the medical and nursing team to restore continence as this is not a very satisfactory arrangement especially if an open wound is also present, e.g. sacral pressure sore, as clearly it is not desirable for these to be contaminated with faeces.

Nocturnal polyuria is a problem in elderly patients (Guite *et al.*, 1988) which is often associated with heavy nocturnal urinary incontinence. Disposable pads are often used when this problem proves to be intractable. This arrangement, however, is not always satisfactory for patients with severe disabilities who need assistance to transfer from bed to a commode or toilet during the night. Use of disposable pads in these patients creates a dilemma for the carer(s) who may have to suffer disturbed sleep to toilet the patient or to change pads. The alternative is to accept that the patient will spend some of the night in a wet bed. A popular alternative management is to use a reusable bed underpad, e.g. a Kylie sheet (see Fig. 37), to contain the nocturnal urinary leakage. These underpads have an absorbent layer, which can absorb up to 2 litres of

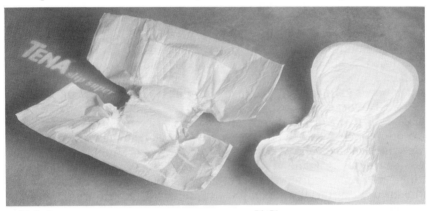

(a) Pads   (b) Diapers

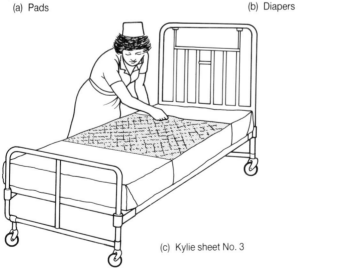

(c) Kylie sheet No. 3

Fig. 37 Examples of an absorbent incontinence pad and diaper which are in common use (courtesy of Mölnlycke Ltd.) plus the reusable bed sheet

urine, under an upper permeable layer. The underpad is placed over a plastic sheet on the patients bed.

Patients sleep on the underpad usually without nightdress or pyjamas. Any urine that leaks during the night is absorbed in the pad which does not feel wet against the patient. The following morning the underpad will need to be laundered but the bed will not be wet and the patient will not have had to lie in a pool of urine. Patients' and carers' quality of life is improved by use of these underpads as there is less need for disturbance of patients' and carers' sleep. The presence of faecal incontinence however precludes their use as faecal contamination of these underpads adversely affects their absorptive capacity.

There are alternative methods of containing heavy intractable urinary incontinence., e.g. sheath urinal or long term catheter linked with a closed urinary drainage system. A device to contain faecal incontinence is also available as an alternative to pads.

The faecal collection device consists of a drainable collecting bag or pouch similar to a colostomy bag (Fig 38). The opening is held in position, over the anus, by a skin protective barrier which adheres to the perianal skin which has to be clean, dry and free from excess hair before the device is applied. The device is applied usually by a nurse with the patient lying on his or her side. The outer margin of the adhesive barrier often needs to be trimmed to make it conform to the shape of the patient's perianal area before it is applied.

The reservoir of the device can accommodate up to 700mls of stool. It should, however, be emptied frequently as its weight when full can pull the device off the perianal skin. When stool is liquid in consistency, drainage is via a tap at the bottom of the reservoir which can be connected to a bedside drainage bag for continuous drainage. Use of this arrangement allows complete containment of faecal leakage thus

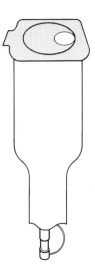

Fig. 38   Example of the faecal collecting bag

reducing the risk of cross infection. The volume of faeces passed can also be recorded.

Solid stool can be drained from the bag by cutting the end of the bag and applying a clamp which can be released as required to empty the bag. This also allows the nursing staff access for the measurement of rectal temperature which is of course the most accurate method of measuring temperature in febrile elderly patients (Downton *et al.*, 1987).

Strapp and Barrett (1988) evaluated the use of this device in the management of 20 faecally incontinent patients aged between 66 and 92 years. All of their patients had a short history of profuse faecal incontinence. Seventeen patients had profuse diarrhoea which was due to gastroenteritis in 15, carcinoma of the rectum in one and ulcerative colitis in the other. Three patients were faecally incontinent following the administration of a potent laxative preparation (Picolax). This had been given as bowel preparation prior to barium enema in one and as treatment of faecal impaction which had been resistant to enemas and other laxative preparations in two patients. Six of the patients evaluated were confused secondary to a dementing illness.

A successful result (complete containment of faecal leakage) was obtained in 18 (90%) of these patients. The failures were due to incorrect application of the device in one patient and the other patient was quite confused and pulled the device off. The accompanying faecal smell was also successfully contained using the device. A reduction in the nursing time and linen requirements for each patient was achieved with a consequent cost saving.

Some patients find the device uncomfortable to wear when they are sitting out of bed in a chair. It is well tolerated by patients who are being nursed in bed.

The device can be left in situ for up to three days and is removed by soaking when it is no longer required or is due to be changed. Strapp and Barrett (1988) found it reduced nursing time, use of bed linen and the surrounding smell in these patients and also helped to maintain their dignity especially in patients with terminal disease.

The indications for use of this device can be considered to be faecal incontinence associated with:

Severe diarrhoea Use of potent laxatives, e.g. during bowel preparation;
Unconsciousness;
Sacral pressure sores;
Bed bound patient;
Terminal illness

The main benefits from use of this device for the terminally ill patient with faecal incontinence are a reduction in any faecal smell due to leakage, fewer turns are required especially if pain control is sub-optimal, and patients can continue to wear their own clothes without the risk of faecal soiling. This device may help patients to achieve the maximal quality of life in the final stages of their illness.

If, despite the above measures, faecal soiling continues then patients and their carers may be grateful for assistance from the incontinence laundry service which most local authority Social Service departments organise. This service can cope with soiled linen without much difficulty. The availability of this service should not, however, encourage health professionals to bypass the assessment and rehabilitation of these patients.

An anal plug (Fig. 39) is currently being developed for use in intractable faecal incontinence to reduce the need for patients to wear pads and/or carry spare underwear.

The initial development of the anal plug took place in Denmark but has since been investigated by Mortensen and Humphreys (1991) in Oxford (UK). Their anal plug is designed to prevent faecal leakage occurring. The ideal plug needs to be easy to insert, effective when postioned in the anus at the level of the anorectal junction and finally easy to remove, especially when there is a desire to defaecate. These plugs are not yet commercially available in the United Kingdom.

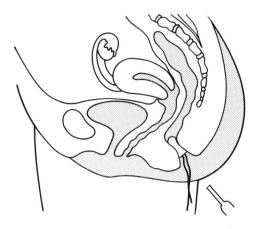

Fig. 39   Example of anal plug placed in the anal canal to prevent faecal leakage

References

Downton JH, Andrews K, Puxty JAH. (1987) 'Silent' pyrexia in the elderly. *Age and and Ageing*; **16**: 41–4.

Guite HF, Bliss MR, Mainwaring-Burton RW, Thomas JM, Drury PL. (1988) Hypothesis: Posture is one of the determinants of the circadian rhythm of urine flow and electrolyte excretion in elderly female patients. *Age and Ageing*; **17**: 241–8.

Mortensen N, Humphreys MS. (1991) The anal continence plug: a disposable device for patients with anorectal incontinence. *Lancet*; **338**: 295–7.

Strapp KJ, Barrett JA. (1988) Unpublished results from a study of the use of a faecal collecting device in a geriatric medical ward in Ladywell Hospital, Salford.

Tobin GW, Brocklehurst JC. (1986) Faecal incontinence in residential homes for the elderly: prevalence, aetiology and management. *Age and Ageing*; **15**: 41–6.

23

Psychological aspects of faecal incontinence in the elderly

LINDA J SMITH AND PAUL S SMITH

Introduction

Though recent years have seen the emergence of an upsurge of interest in urinary incontinence in the elderly, a trawl through the psychological literature on elimination problems highlights the as yet sad lack of interest specifically in the problem of faecal incontinence. Many recent studies of elimination disorders in the elderly have looked at incidence rates, aetiology, attitudes and psychological effects. Others have begun to look at the effects of continence retraining programmes. Yet, at best, incontinence of the bowel is referred to only in passing, while many studies reporting on 'incontinence' actually only refer to urinary incontinence. Thus, any discussion of the problem of faecal incontinence in the elderly must at present draw heavily on studies on urinary incontinence in the elderly and faecal incontinence in other age groups.

The whole size and nature of the problem is at first glance depressing and it is certainly so for elderly people as well as their carers. Incontinence is often seen as an inevitable consequence of both normal and abnormal ageing processes. It is often viewed as a specific symptom of organic disorders, for example, within dementia, and it is often viewed as intractable. In this chapter, we shall consider whether these views are justified. In relation to treatment, it is argued here that recent evidence warrants a better balance between physical and psychological approaches. A psychological approach does not deny a biological component to a problem and the work described by Ehrmann (1983) and Whitehead *et al.* (1984, 1985), as well as many other, more recent publications, are good examples of this.

The personal and emotional experience of being incontinent

Urinary incontinence, for example has been described as a source of 'appreciable morbidity' (Macauley *et al.*, 1987), as a distressing, socially disabling condition (Simons, 1985; Wyman *et al.*, 1990), likely to result in 'negative psychological and physical affects . . .' (Yu, 1987) and which can, in the elderly, make the difference between dependence and independence. There is widespread acceptance in the literature of loss of self-esteem and self-confidence, physical and psychological decline and social disengagement.

Clearly, the only people who really know what it is like to lose control of the continence process are incontinence sufferers themselves. Sadly, many elderly people suffering from severe dementia and whose general functioning has deteriorated are unable to articulate and describe the experience. Some ten years ago, however, a few personal accounts of the experience and surveys of the views and experiences of incontinent people began to emerge, highlighting the importance of practical matters in coping with incontinence in a continent society, as well as with the behaviour and attitudes of others (Borthwick, 1985; Masham, 1985). From such accounts, it is clear that a high degree of competence and practice is necessary for those who use continence aids, as is strong motivation, a sense of humour and a firm routine. All this is necessary to deal with what most of us take for granted. Gartley and her colleagues (Balson *et al.*, 1985; Gartley and Humpal, 1984) give qualitative descriptions from open-ended interviews with a range of incontinence sufferers. Feelings of anger, shame, depression, isolation, fear of accidents and changes in feelings about sexuality were highly salient, recurrent themes. Wheelchair users were reported to rate the re-establishment of control over continence processes more highly than regaining control over their legs! Gartly and Humpal describe coming to terms with incontinence as a progression through a series of stages moving from depression to anger, to a final philosophical and tolerant view of their own incontinence and others' responses to it and them.

Such reports of the psychological effects of incontinence as were contained in these highly personal accounts resulted in a widespread belief in a substantial impact of incontinence on mental well-being, social relationships and daily living activities. Valuable as they were in raising social awareness of a problem affecting substantial numbers of people, such studies nevertheless suffered from methodological shortcomings. More recently, however, surveys have begun to assess in a more objective way the psychosocial impact of incontinence on incontinent individuals and their carers by studying the statistical relationships between factors such as type and severity of incontinence and various measures of mental well-being (Wyman *et al.*,

1987; Wyman *et al.*, 1990; Mitteness, 1990; Jeter and Wagner, 1990; Ouslander and Abelson, 1990; Norton *et al.*, 1990). These studies do, indeed, show that a proportion of sufferers experience restrictions in daily living activities as well as social embarrassment, shame, lower self-esteem, etc. However, the picture now emerging is by no means as simple as might have been expected from the early accounts. Despite some difficulties in comparing findings across studies, two findings do emerge consistently from the literature. Firstly, the majority of sufferers either do not come forward, or delay substantially in coming forward to seek help from the services (Norton *et al.*, 1988). Secondly, the majority of sufferers perceive the problem as a nuisance rather than a serious problem (Wyman *et al.*, 1987; Wyman *et al.*, 1990; Ouslander and Abelson, 1990; Simons, 1985; Jeter and Wagner, 1990). This is not to deny the incontinence is associated with significant mental health symptoms for a minority of incontinent individuals (Macauley *et al.*, 1987, 1991). However, it is interesting to note that mental well-being, however measured, seems to be unrelated to measures of frequency and in some studies, severity of incontinence (Wyman *et al.*, 1987). Thus, some individuals experience substantial ill effects disproportionate to the objective severity of the problem. As Wyman *et al.* (1990) state, there would appear to be 'wide variability in response to urinary incontinence'. As physical ill-health has been linked to mental ill health (Herzog *et al.*, 1988) and incontinent people tend to have more physical health problems and poorer health status (Palmer, 1988), physical ill health cannot be ruled out as the factor in many studies responsible for the decrease in mental well-being, self-esteem, life satisfaction, etc. Additionally, physical ill health tends to increase with age. Finally, some of those who do experience a severe reaction to incontinence may have been predisposed to do so by personality characteristics such as high anxiety.

If the majority of incontinence sufferers are, after all, not substantially affected in a negative way by their problem, it is tempting to speculate that this may be *one* of the reasons why approximately 50–70% of sufferers fail to come forward to receive help. In fact, there is some support from the literature for this hypothesis: among reasons given for not seeking help, a sizable proportion of sufferers gave the reason 'not important enough' (British Association of Continence Care, 1991; Simons, 1985).

Personality, mental health and faecal incontinence

Terminology

Before proceeding further, a brief discussion on the terminology used in this chapter will be necessary to avoid confusion. The reader will notice throughout the interchangeable use of the terms 'soiling', 'encopresis' and 'faecal incontinence'. This does, in fact, reflect the use in the psychological literature of different terms by different authors when referring to the same phenomenon. Though the terms faecal incontinence, faecal soiling and encopresis have implied a distinction of some validity between different types of bowel incontinence, in practice such a distinction between disorders of organic origin or functional origin is, as we shall see, becoming increasingly unclear. Advances in knowledge are resulting in definitions of encopresis that reflect both physiological and psychological factors so that the definitions no longer reflect the historical dichtomy of organic versus psychogenic encopresis.

Furthermore, later discussion will seek to demonstrate that a distinction between faecal incontinence of organic or psychogenic origin may also ultimately be found to have less validity in terms of *treatment* than was originally thought to be the case, as faecal incontinence and constipation of organic origin can be successfully treated with a variety of psychological techniques. Finally, it is clear that abnormal measures of bowel function may persist despite clinically successful treatment for severe constipation and soiling (Loening-Baucke, 1984a, 1984b).

What then is the effect, if any, of faecal incontinence on mental well-being? Though no studies appear to have addressed specifically the question of the impact of faecal incontinence on the mental well-being of the adult sufferer, some studies have looked at the relationship between mental health or personality and soiling in children. Whatever the effects of urinary incontinence on the individual, one might intuitively expect the effects of faecal incontinence to be more devastating. Faecal incontinence must rank as one of the most potentially humiliating problems a person can experience: whereas it is possible, though often difficult, for a sufferer of urinary incontinence to conceal the problem, it is rarely possible for an encopretic person to do so, with the result that he or she may become a virtual social outcast. In relation to children, parents have been found to be less tolerant of faecal incontinence than of nocturnal enuresis (Doleys *et al.*, 1981). Small wonder, then, that the work on encopretic children, for example, finds some evidence of emotional disturbance, for as well as the effect on peer relationships, encopretic children may suffer physical abuse by parents (Schaeffer, 1979; Vidailhet, 1983). As health and social services become stretched and the burden of care falls increasingly and often relentlessly on stressed families, abuse of elderly, dependent people is likely to become an area of increasing concern. Although no studies have as yet emerged to show how far incontinence of urine and/or faeces may contribute to physical abuse, Yu and Kaltreider (1987) have studied the effects on residential care staff of caring long term for those incontinent of urine. They have demonstrated that healthcare providers can experience considerable stress, apparently due to dealing with incontinence.

Psycho-analytic sources point to a supposed high rate of personality disturbances in encopretics (Vidailhet, 1983). Elderly sufferers would be regarded as having regressed to infancy. Support for such claims come mainly from early case studies of psycho-analyis and uncontrolled, retrospective studies. More recent studies have attempted to adopt a more scientific approach to the question of whether there are indeed differences between encopretic and non-encopretic children; if so, what is the nature of any differences; and what is the relationship between the symptom of encopresis and the personality characteristics or mental health problems. Again, it is difficult to compare findings directly across studies. Basically, however, the findings are similar to those for urinary incontinence; although a proportion of encopretic children may have behaviour or mental health problems, these are not as severe as those found in non-encopretic children referred for mental health services, with the behaviour of most encopretic children falling within the normal range (Gabel *et al.*, 1986; Friman *et al.*, 1988; Stark *et al.*, 1990). Thus, the vast majority of encopretic children do not have serious emotional or behavioural problems, though there is little doubt that self-esteem is lower (Stark *et al.*, 1990) and peer relationships as well as positive feelings about life may be affected (Owens-Stively, 1987; Landman *et al.*, 1986). Such differences as are found are probably mainly the result of the encopresis (e.g. Gabel *et al.*, 986) as opposed to the cause, with any mild problems of anxiety, unhappiness, inhibition, etc. tending to disappear with successful treatment.

Psychological approaches to the treatment of faecal incontinence

Some interesting surveys on urinary incontinence have sought information about sufferers' intuitive methods for coping with their problems, such as fluid restriction, use of pads, location of toilets in advance, or avoidance of places with restricted toilet access (British Association of Continence Care, 1991; Norton *et al.*, 1988; Jeter and Wagner, 1990). No similar information is available for sufferers of faecal incontinence, though some people with a strong gastrocolic reflex avoid eating prior to or during outings. As with urinary incontinence, a substantial proportion of sufferers of bowel problems probably fail to seek help (Thomson and Heaton, 1980; Sandler *et al.*, 1984). For those who do, abdominal pain (Sandler *et al.*, 1984) and soiling (Drossman *et al.*, 1986) are significant factors.

In the psychological literature, treatment approaches have variously subclassified faecal incontinence according to whether it is primary or secondary, organic or functional (often also referred to as idiopathic or psychogenic), retentive or non-retentive. The validity of these distinctions in relation to treatment and its effectiveness, is, however, unclear. With respect to the primary versus secondary distinction, such evidence as is available seems to indicate that secondary faecal incontinence is amenable to the same range of psychological techniques as primary encopresis. As we shall see later on, the distinction between organic and functional soiling is not necessarily a clearcut one as far as treatment approaches are concerned. Biofeedback and other training techniques from psychology have been used with success in people with diagnosed organic disorders of bowel function as well as those with abnormal physiological responses but without demonstrable organic disorders. Furthermore, though clear physiological differences in bowel function have been found between 'normal' subjects and those with constipation, faecal impaction or faecal incontinence (Loening-Baucke, 1984a, 1984b), such differences may remain even after successful bowel retraining.

Finally, perhaps the most frequently used of these distinctions is that of retentive versus non-retentive encopresis. It has been agreed that the vast majority of encopretic people suffer to some extent from constipation (Doleys *et al.*, 1981). Certainly, constipation is a major factor in faecal incontinence in long-stay institutional populations, such as the elderly, the mentally ill and people with a mental handicap. Many factors which have an effect on constipation, such as fibre insufficiency, reduced fluid intake, reduce mobility, overuse of artificial aids to defaecation, reduced abdominal and intestinal muscle tone, psychological factors such as anxiety and depression, together with many common medications, are all to be found in the elderly (Resnick, 1985) as well as in other high dependency populations. As we shall see, however, the same range of behavioural techniques has been successfully applied to both constipated and non-constipated faecally incontinent patients, though some studies have combined behavioural techniques with the use of artificial aids to evacuation over a limited period of time.

Assessment

Obtaining a reliable and objective 'baseline' record of a problem, behaviour, whilst standard practice in behavioural psychology, has in the past been less frequently a part of routine clinical practice in some other disciplines. The importance of such a record before beginning on any programme of behavioural change cannot be overstated. The unreliability of subjective estimates of incontinence has been highlighted, for example, by Blackwell (1990) in a study of nocturnal enuresis in children, Smith (1979) for incontinence among institutionalised residents with a mental handicap, and Turner *et al.* (1988) and Sabin (1990) for faecal incontinence within institutional care settings for the elderly with dementia. It is hard to imagine how there can be differences in ratings for a phenomenon such as faecal incontinence, but human judgements of human behaviour are fallible and affected by a number of factors. Firstly, subjective estimates and reports typically overestimate the frequency and/or severity of a problem behaviour: stressed carers can be substantially subjectively influenced in their reports according to the situation around the time of reporting. Secondly, shift systems in any care establishment are a source of unreliability, with some staff being more observant than others, as well as handling problems in a different way. Thirdly, an objective record can serve to highlight easily remedied environmental factors. Finally, elderly people are not necessarily reliable even when capable of providing estimates of their own problems (Whitehead *et al.*, Donald *et al.*, 1985).

Objective recording can provide information about possible deterioration over time as well as the opportunity to evaluate the effectiveness of intervention. Resnick (1985) summarises important factors for assessment as follows: medical and family history, food and fluid intake, medications, daily activities, emotional state, present medical state, toilet habits. Toilet habits, including frequency, consistency and amount of both continent or incontinent episodes, are more reliably recorded on individually daily record forms than in general daily record books or patients' case notes, with each entry signed by the staff member responsible for care at that time. There is also a need to identify which component in the toileting sequence the client is unable to, or has difficulty, completing (Brown and Doolan, 1983; Holden and Woods, 1982). This includes ability to handle clothes and find the way to the toilet as well as the ability to perform appropriately on the toilet.

General environmental effects

If bowel function is viewed predominently as a biological mechanism of waste control, it may seem strange at first glance that external factors can be claimed to exert an influence. At this point, there- fore, we will briefly outline some evidence which strongly suggests that environmental factors can indeed significantly influence bowel control. In the general population, factors such as diet, toilet design and posture may be relevant. In groups more vulnerable to problems of bowel control, such as institutionalised elderly people with dementia or severe mental handicaps, evidence points also to the influence of carers and the general quality of the surroundings.

Diet and posture

That the legacy of a refined diet is constipation and straining to defaecate is increasingly accepted. That the legacy of Western toilet design is also undesirable has been less well documented, though suspicion is high. One of the few architects and designers to have considered this seriously is Kira (1976). Why the high pedestal toilet evolved in Western Europe is unclear. It is certainly unnatural. Sitting to defaecate, as if quite literally on a throne, allows neither gravity nor the appropriate muscle groups to operate effectively. The natural human posture for defaecation is the squat posture, which allows increased intra-abdominal pressure while straightening the lower end of the colon. The increasing practice of some Third World countries of forsaking the squat toilet for the Western pedestal toilet is to be deplored. Anecdotal evidence suggests physical dangers for elderly people in addition to increased constipation and straining. Stories of people from rural districts in developing countries encountering modern pedestal toilets for the first time in city department stores tell of injuries caused by mistaken attempts to squat on the pedestal toilet. Less than steady elderly people, in particular, may topple off their dizzy perch! Far from exporting our toileting practices to the rest of the world, the implication for our more 'advanced' society is that the toilet seat should be low enough for the feet to rest firmly on the floor so that some flexion of the thighs is possible. If this is not the case, then something placed below the toilet on which to rest the feet may help facilitate the passing of faeces.

Space and living conditions

Studies on clinical groups, particularly the hospitalised elderly and those with a mental handicap, illustrate other effects of environment on toileting behaviour. Hereford *et al*. (1973) found evidence that reducing overcrowding, increasing space and demarcating territory reduced wetting and soiling in a group of institutionalised profoundly mentally handicapped men. In a larger study of 200 hospitalised mentally handicapped residents, Duker (1983) found that size of living group and access to toilet were significantly related to bladder control. Without the introduction of any additional continence training or treatment programmes, Shrubsole and Smith (1984) found a 30% reduction in the frequency of incontinence after upgrading of an overcrowded, impoverished ward to provide increased living space and better general living conditions for a group of institutionalised mentally handicapped adults.

Of what relevance is this to bowel problems in elderly people? Similarities exist particularly with respect to institutionalised residental populations. People with a mental handicap have in the past been regarded as having intractable, untreatable incontinence, yet their toileting behaviours have been found to be substantially affected by environmental effects. Sadly, at a time when institutional populations of mentally handicapped people are decreasing, thus permitting improved environmental conditions, pressure to admit elderly people to institutional beds is increasing.

Access to toilets, mobility and confusion

Most people understand obvious inadequacies in toilet facilities, such as lack of wheelchair access. Here, minimum standards are easily set for door width and minimum working space. When these standards are not met, it is relatively easy to assess and condemn this state of affairs. Much less attention is paid to setting measurable standards for other aspects of toilet access for elderly confused people. Nevertheless, the evidence suggests that physical environment often militates against continence in this client group, both at home and in residential care settings.

Let us look first at obstacles in the way of elderly people with faecal incontinence. Noelker (1987) surveyed a large community sample of cognitively impaired elderly people with and without incontinence. Both those suffering from urinary incontinence alone and those with combined faecal and urinary incontinence were found to have a significantly higher number of 'navigational barriers' in the home, such as stairs, absence of railings, bathroom fittings difficult to use.

Two recent unpublished studies of elderly people in UK long stay, psychogeriatric hospital settings have also raised cause for concern in this respect. The first (Turner *et al.*, 1988) reported 24% of a population of over 1000 patients to be faecally incontinent during the day. Yet in some instances the distances between living areas and the toilets were as much as 36 metres. The second report (Sabin, 1990) found distances from living to toilet areas ranging from 10 to 58 metres! In order to look at the association between incontinence and navigational barriers, Sabin viewed the floor plans of the living accommodation in terms of choice points in a maze learning task. Each time a decision had to be made about direction en route to toilet, this was scored as a choice point. There was a highly significant statistical relationship between increased choice points and increased number of patients with urinary or faecal incontinence.

If access to toilets were easier, would it make any real difference? The answer is well illustrated by Holden and Woods (1982) in an observational study of eight incontinence women suffering from senile dementia. Direct observation showed that five of them had difficulty in finding the toilet at the right time, but could use the toilet appropriately once there. From a behavioural point of view, continence is not a simple process, but involves a complex set of component skills (Smith and Smith, 1987). Mental factors such as confusion or disorientation, as well as impaired mobility or other motor skills deficits, can interfere with this set of skills. Apart from structural changes to the environment to improve toilet proximity and access, such as providing fire doors which remain open but close automatically on activation of the alarm, there are a number of simple changes to the physical environment to provide cues to toilet finding for elderly confused people in residential settings. These include signing toilet routes and leaving toilet doors open so that their function is more clearly seen. Some toilet doors in institutional settings have unnecessary spring mechanisms which make them shut automatically. Doors should be colour coded to contrast rather than blend with the general decor. Colours at the red end of the spectrum are generally easier for older people to detect, as perception of the colour red has been shown to fade least with age (Turner *et al.*, 1988). There is at present little hard evidence of the effectiveness of environmental cueing on the toileting behaviour of confused elderly people, but its effectiveness in other areas of retraining for the elderly is well documented. Though highly valued by staff in hospital settings, such procedures help facilitate the process of maintaining continence.

Finally, Panella (1986) believes that cognitively impaired individuals still recognise bowel and bladder signals, but ambulant impaired people may have difficulty finding the toilet, undressing, performing appropriately and redressing, in order to remain independent. As well as being easily accessible and provided with aids for people with handicaps, he feels bathrooms should otherwise be as bare as possible, with distractions kept to a minimum. Smith and Smith (1987), however, do not entirely agree with Panella's views on the necessity of a barren, distraction-free environment. People with a mental handicap have precisely the same difficulties in perceiving relevant environmental cues. However, recognition of cues in toilet training programmes for people with a profound degree of mental handicap can be successfully taught using behavioural techniques such as backward chaining or shaping. In contrast to Panella, Smith and Smith attempt to make toilet areas more comfortable and attractive for trainer and patient.

The psycho-analytic approach

From a practical point of view, psycho-analysis has made little contribution to the treatment of faecal incontinence and therefore need not be seriously considered here. The limited number of case studies to be found are unimpressive both in terms of methodology and results, with baseline, treatment and follow up data either inadequate or in most cases completely lacking. Treatment times reported are lengthy by comparison with other methods of treatment, with most case studies involving children within the normal range of intelligence, so that spontaneous remission cannot be ruled out. Many successful behavioural interventions report on previous unsuccessful psycho-analytic involvement.

Behavioural approaches to treatment

Though behavioural approaches to the treatment of urinary and faecal incontinence have been in increasing use since the 1960s, the quality of intervention studies on the subject of faecal incontinence varies markedly from those on urinary incontinence, the former being largely restricted to single case studies or small groups of case studies. Such analyses as those, for example, carried out into the relative effectiveness of the different components in standard treatment approaches to nocturnal enuresis (Bollard and Nettlebeck, 1982) are virtually absent for faecal incontinence. To overcome the limitations inherent in single case studies, a number of authors have applied reversal designs (Rolider and van Houten, 1985; Sanavio, 1981; Bornstein *et al.*, 1983). Lyon (1984), though, feels a return to baseline conditions is highly questionable after a period of successful treatment for such a distressing problem as faecal incontinence. This may indeed be a particular problem for patients who have suffered from severe and longstanding faecal impaction, with all the attendant risks. Studies using control groups can also be found (Berg *et al.*, 1983; Rovetto, 1979). Other authors have begun to compare the effectivenesss of different factors in treatment (Houts and Peterson, 1986; Houts *et al.*, 1988; O'Brien *et al.*, 1986). Most of the studies quoted here have involved people with a mental handicap or children.

Approaches to the treatment of encopresis have variously used rewards for appropriate toilet use and/or for clean underwear; 'extinction' (ignoring), 'time out from reward' (withdrawing of rewards or the opportunity to earn these for a specified period of time), 'response cost' (fining), or a range of more aversive consequences such as 'correction' (rectifying the situation, e.g. through washing soiled underwear), 'overcorrection' (restoring the situation to better than the original state, for example by washing out soiled pants plus three other items, or washing soiled pants for 20 minutes), or 'positive practice' (practising the steps of appropriate toilet behaviour, such as going to the toilet and back a specified number of times from different parts of the house) for soiling. Reward and punishment techniques may be used in combination. Additionally, a behavioural approach has often been combined with the use of medication on a temporary basis, a more permanent change in diet, or the use of bulking agents. Finally, treatments have been applied on both an inpatient and an outpatient basis. At present, the choice of which of the above techniques to use is largely a matter for clinical intuition.

Use of rewards only

No papers report on the exclusive use of punishments. However, a number of papers report the successful use of reward procedures only. Some (Knell and Moore, 1990; Berrigan and Stedman, 1989; Berg *et al.*, 1983; Bulkely and Sahami, 1983; Bornstein *et al.*, 1983), reward both clean underwear and bowel movements passed into the toilet, while others reward only bowel movements in the toilet (Houts and Peterson, 1986; Brown and Doolan, 1983; Bach and Moylan, 1975; Kaplan, 1985). Some authors feel intuitively that rewards for clean underwear should never be used where constipation and faecal impaction are factors, as the patient may withhold faeces further in an attempt to remain clean. Rewards used have included stars, tokens, money, edibles, as well as exclusive carer time. Studies have involved patients with and without faecal retention (though many studies fail to provide information on this) as well as those of different ages. There is therefore some difficulty in comparing results. However, reported treatment times using rewards for bowel movements in the toilet only seem on the face of it to be little different from those where rewards were administered additionally for clean underwear, being approximately 13 to 25 weeks for the former and 13 to 20 for the latter. Thus, there would seem to be little evidence to suggest that the use of rewards for clean underwear poses a general risk for those suffering from constipation although the occasional case may be noted (Knell and Moore, 1990). On the other hand, Kaplan (1985) reports on a study involving 32 children using rewards for toilet use only and Berg *et al.* (1983) on 40 children where both cleanliness and toilet use were rewarded: success rates were similar for both groups, with a 20–30% failure rate. Thus, the additional staff time involved in carrying out clean underwear checks several times daily may not be cost effective.

Use of rewards and aversive consequences

The majority of papers report on the combined use of rewards for appropriate toilet use and/or cleanliness, together with some form of punishment for soiling accidents. Again, some authors believe punishment should not be used in cases where constipation and faecal impaction are an issue. Other authors express serious misgivings regarding the use of aversive techniques due to their potential for abuse (Lyon, 1984). This is a view with which the present authors have great sympathy. The theoretical rationale behind some of these practices, such as correction, overcorrection and positive practice, is at best unclear and their use is therefore regarded by some as ethically questionable (Pfadt and Sullivan, 1980). Many programmes which require the patient to wash soiled clothing, (correction) often refer to this practice specifically as 'educative', as 'taking responsibility' (Plachetta, 1976; Davis *et al.*, 1976, 1977; Dawson *et al.*, 1990), or as 'logical consequences' (Lyon, 1984). Authors may even state categorically that the procedure was not intended as a punishment. However, whether washing soiled clothes by hand, possibly in cold water, is perceived as educative or punishing, depends not on the trainer's perceptions but on those of the trainee, the latter depending substantially on his or her level of cognitive functioning. Thus, younger children and severely cognitively impaired adults are unlikely to have the necessary concepts of responsibility either fully developed or, in the case of the elderly or the mentally handicapped, remaining intact and will almost certainly find the practice to be punishing. Similarly, the practice of overcorrection, where the individual is required to restore the situation to better than the original state, has been viewed as highly punishing (Pfadt and Sullivan, 1980). The procedure of positive practice, where the patient must complete the appropriate toileting sequence a specified number of times after each episode of incontinence, has been deemed to involve a substantial element of fatigue and hence must be regarded as punishing.

There is a clear expectation in ethical guidelines that, where punishment techniques are used, a hierarchy of least drastic alternatives should be tried, and that the emphasis in any programme must always be heavily on the reward side. Additionally, research into learning has established that learning is faster under conditions of reward than of punishment. Sadly, punishment procedures often seem to attract more staff interest than reward procedures. Kolko (1989), for example, states that the consistency with which various elements of a programme was carried out was highest for the 'clean up procedure' (unspecified), with less consistency for rewards for appropriate toilet use, prompted toileting trips often forgotten and pants checking procedures abandoned due to staff non-compliance. Some programmes have used punishment procedures only as an added feature if rewards did not eliminate the problem (Bosch, 1988; Stark *et al.*, 1990; O'Brien *et al.*, 1986). Other studies appear in effect to have emphasised the soiling exclusively by punishing soiling and rewarding clean underwear, with no apparent attempt to build up appropriate toilet use (Foxx, 1985; Davis *et al.*, 1976; Ayllon *et al.*, 1975). Studies combining the use of rewards and punishments report a wide range of treatment times from two days to 14 weeks. On the fact of it at least, treatment times would therefore appear to be shorter for programmes using a combination of rewards and punishments. Thus, though some authors believe constipation to be an important factor for consideration in any treatment programme (Kaplan, 1985), in practice a substantial number of clinicians seem to disregard it completely, with around 50% of studies not specifying whether patients were constipated or not. Again on the face of it, the use of aversive consequences for soiling would not appear to aggravate constipation by causing further retention.

Some studies have carried out treatment on an inpatient basis, either initially or entirely, for cases regarded as more difficult or in order to ensure greater control over training procedures (Webster and Gore, 1980; Kolko, 1989; Steege and Harper, 1989). Unfortunately, it is not possible with such a small number of studies to make any sort of comparison of treatment times for inpatient versus outpatient treatment. Admission to hospital is, however, likely to be fairly traumatic for the client groups who more typically suffer from faecal incontinence. Treatment can almost always be carried out successfully in the community in the experience of the present authors, even with more disabled clients. What is clear, though, is that a very substantial degree of support and monitoring is required, including a home-based trainer in the most difficult cases.

Despite the relatively smaller number of studies on behavioural treatments of faecal incontinence compared with those for urinary incontinence, the available evidence indicates that an intensive, structured behavioural approach is highly effective. A combination of rewards and punishments may be used, but clinicians working with the elderly with cognitive impairment may prefer to use rewards only, or to add mild punishments (such as a sharp reprimand) only where the use of rewards alone has failed to completely eliminate the problem. The purpose of any punishment procedure is not retribution but to help the individual to learn to differentiate between appropriate and inappropriate behaviour. As such, the minimum level of punishment necessary to achieve this purpose is used. Rewards and punishments should be administered immediately upon performance of the behaviour in order to be effective: rewarding a person with severe cognitive impairment five or ten minutes after passing urine or faeces into the toilet will have no effect on the behaviour. Staff often show a basic dislike of using primary reinforcers (reinforcers based on a primary biological drive, such as food or drink) as rewards over and above praise. However, in practice it is clear that the use of a variety of drinks or small edibles speeds up the learning process. Primary reinforcers are easily phased out at the end of training, though this must always be done gradually to reduce the risk of relapse. Edibles can include the use of savouries or segments of fruit as well as sweet items.

Other factors in training programmes

Medication

Doleys (1978) has suggested that treatments employing purgatives, laxatives and suppositories seem 'doomed to fail because they provide no mechanism for the development and maintenance of appropriate toileting skill'. Indeed, some case studies refer to previous treatment failures which used only regular clear-outs or laxative use in an attempt to 'retrain' the bowel, but where bowel movements ceased upon cessation of medication. Without the inclusion of a specific learning framework, it is indeed hard to see how the bowel could be expected to become 'retrained' solely by means of regular use of medication, which is believed by many to result in 'lazy bowel' syndrome. The majority of studies using medication have done so in the context of a programme based clearly on psychological learning theory. Some studies have used mineral oil or milk of magnesia to ensure the occurrence of the behaviour to be rewarded as well as to prevent impaction. Enemas or suppositories may be used as an initial method of clearing impacted faeces, often in combination with subsequent laxative use. Additionally, suppositories and enemas have also been used to act as a 'discriminative stimulus' for toilet sitting by increasing the appropriate sensation for defaecation.

Attempts to enhance the predefaecation urge would seem appropriate in cases of constipated people with diminished perception of the urge to evacuate. Kaplan (1985) argues that the use of enemas and suppositories is in fact more appropriate than that of laxatives. A more carefully timed urge to defaecate is probably easier to achieve using these, thus permitting the urge to be reconditioned to a more normally occurring environmental event such as the ingestion of food. Indeed, one unusual study by Rovetto (1979) used suppositories in just this way to successfully recondition the urge to defaecate in a group of housewives with chronic constipation. The urge was conditioned to a time of day of their choice when they could guarantee to sit down with a cup of coffee and a newspaper. In this way, classical conditioning to the coffee and newspaper occurred, but only for the time of day of original training. This is a novel application of a classical conditioning paradigm which appears to have been given little attention in the literature but which would seem to have great potential due to the ease of administration. Recent experience in teaching a woman with a severe degree of mental handicap has shown that this technique can be used to successfully condition the urge to defaecate to the ingestion of breakfast. If it is true that elderly people with cognitive impairment retain recognition of bowel and bladder cues (Panella, 1986), then the urge to defaecate could be reconditioned in this group in just this way. Rovetto used a cup of coffee and the reading of a newspaper as the conditioned stimulus. In an institutional setting, meals would be a more appropriate conditioned stimulus, as mealtimes are usually highly reliable and stable temporal events. The only additional work for staff would involve the administration of a suppository immediately before breakfast and toileting afterwards. Medication to increase the urge to defaecate has usually, though not always, been used in conjunction with 'stimulus control' (prompted toilet sitting). This should hopefully increase the 'hit' rate on the toilet thus increasing the opportunity for rewards and speeding up learning of the appropriate behaviour. Most studies use a toilet sit of up to ten minutes. Medication is usually phased out gradually during training.

Diet and fibre

The use of suppositories or enemas as a discriminative stimulus in the context of a structured programme based on psychological learning theories would seem in theory reasonable. Other studies have used increased fibre in the diet or bulking agents such as Fybogel to produce a discriminative stimulus in a more natural way. Clearly, where possible, this approach would be more desirable. Though many studies have added bulk to the diet in conjunction with the use of operant conditioning techniques (Houts and Peterson, 1986), it is clear that the addition of bulk in the diet together with stimulus control (prompted toilet sitting) alone can effect success for some patients without necessarily including rewards and/or punishments (Houts *et al.*, 1988). However, diet is often difficult to change in a sufficiently major way as to have much effect. Bran may be added to the food as an alternative, but the effects of bran are not simple, depending on the type used and how it has been processed prior to ingestion (Heaton, 1990). Additionally, some authors do not recommend high fibre diets for immobile or elderly patients (Donald *et al.*, 1985), as high residue diets have been implicated in sigmoid volvulus, a disease of the aged or mentally disabled (Rosenthal and Marshall, 1987). Others, though, have successfully used bran to relieve constipation in physically and mentally handicapped patients (Lupson and Walton, 1981). Larger doses of bulk forming agents may be necessary to achieve the same effects in a disabled population than in normal, healthy, younger subjects (Fischer *et al.*, 1985; Liebel *et al.*, 1990). Finally, the addition of large amounts of bulk to the diet, in whatever form, is not without risk: phytobezoars, though uncommon, have occurred in institutionalised people or those suffering from mental illness (Sroujieh, 1988).

Although caution must be exercised in the use of increased fibre or bulking agents, benefits have been obtained in their use with severely disabled people. Certainly, increased fibre can be used to good effect in the context of a structured behavioural programme where careful monitoring can be ensured. Clearly, careful monitoring is required.

Stimulus control and the gastrocolic reflex

Prompted toilet sitting (stimulus control), usually for up to ten minutes, is often though not always used at times when the urge to defaecate would be expected to occur naturally. For most people, the urge to defaecate occurs once per day, usually in the morning after breakfast. However, as the urge for others may also occur after any meal, or indeed after each meal, prompted toilet sits should be scheduled to occur after each meal until such time as a pattern of defaecation begins to re-emerge. Patterns of defaecation are often impossible to identify in people suffering from chronic constipation and faecal impaction. The use of normal physiological response patterns in retraining is clearly important. Unfortunately, while it would be normal for nurses to prompt patients to toilet after meals, it is clear from the literature that many psychologists are unaware of the importance of this reflex and may schedule toiletings for times at which defaecation would not normally be expected to occur. The importance of combining stimulus control with the gastrocolic reflex would seem obvious when suppositories, bulking agents or increased fibre are used to increase the predefaecation urge. In this way, the urge can then be classically conditioned or reconditioned to the most natural stimulus of all, namely that of sitting, on the toilet after meals.

Reasons for failure

Approximately 70% of cases of faecal incontinence treated using behavioural techniques are said to be cured or markedly improved at one year follow up (Kaplan, 1985; Berg *et al.*, 1983; Bosch, 1988; Dawson *et al.*, 1990). Despite this, some authors continue to describe faecal incontinence as being difficult to treat (Steege and Harper, 1989). What is clear is that, despite the success of behavioural approaches in the majority of cases, around 30% of cases remain intractable (Landman *et al.*, 1983; Berg *et al.*, 1983). Why this should be is not understood though a number of studies have begun to address this issue. Landman *et al.* (1983) believe that potential causes of failure might include as yet unrecognised physical differences, mental health problems, or non-compliance. However, using a behavioural approach, Kaplan (1985) successfully treated eight out of 11 children with significant family or mental health problems. Of significance, failure was also unrelated either to level of intellectual functioning or diagnosed neurological involvement, a finding supported by other studies. Stark *et al.* (1990) studied management and coping styles in parents of encopretic children. No differences were found except in compliance with the programme. Levine and Bakow (1976) and Stark *et al.* (1990) similarly report greater failure to comply amongst treatment failures, in particular with the administration of enemas and suppositories.

Steege and Harper (1989) suggest that the 'acceptability' of a pro-posed programme (i.e. the consumer's or the carer's understanding of it and of its effectiveness) is crucial to compliance. They ensured that effectiveness could be demonstrated by carrying out the treatment on an inpatient basis before expecting carers to carry out the programme at home. Berg *et al.* (1983) likewise recommend inpatient treatment for those with a history of failure and Stark *et al.* (1990) also feel that some families may not possess the necessary skills to follow a demanding treatment regime consistently. However, previously suc-cessful inpatient treatment does not guarantee compliance by carers with maintenance procedures (Goldstein *et al.*, 1969). The present authors have found a high level of support and supervision to be essential to ensure compliance. Daily support may be necessary in the initial stages of a programme, reducing to once a week when success is becoming apparent, and then gradually phasing out during the maintenance period. Failure to comply is a well established problem even for the maintenance of a previously successful programme. It is almost certainly a key factor in initial success of a programme.

Continence training specifically with the elderly or elderly confused

What of continence retraining specifically with the elderly or elderly confused? What evidence is there for effectiveness, and indeed cost effectiveness, of training with these groups? Though some programmes have sought to retrain both bowel and bladder continence, few give data specifically for faecal incontinence and almost all relate only to bladder retraining. In this respect, somewhat confusing to the British reader is the fact that many American studies refer to 'soiled' underclothes or pads when they appear to mean 'wet'.

Early attempts to retrain continence in the elderly with dementia are discussed by Burgio *et al.* (1988). These tended to concentrate on rewarding dry clothing but not appropriate elimination on the toilet and did not produce promising results. Early studies with cognitively intact elderly people reported greater success and included the use of praise, social interaction, tokens, sweets, cigarettes, and meals for dryness and/or appropriate elimination, and some aversive consequences (Burgio *et al.*, 1988). More recent studies have looked at continence retraining in both elderly confused and elderly cognitively intact people, as well as the non-ambulant or physically heavily dependent. For example, Pinkston *et al.* (1987) studied the effect of prompted voiding and reinforcement on three non-ambulant, cognitively impaired, high dependency women between 77 and 94 years old. Using a multiple baseline design, a very thorough baseline recording procedure was implemented followed by a training programme consisting of two-hourly dryness checks together with two-hourly toileting. Wetness was ignored, dryness praised and appropriate passing of urine in the toilet was detected with litmus paper and rewarded with snacks, as were spontaneous requests for the toilet. All three patients showed a systematic and substantial decrease in incontinence with training. Though training increased the number of occasions on which patients were toileted by staff during the training period over the baseline period, patients actually spent less time sitting on the toilet. There is, however, difficulty in determining whether the reduction in incontinence was due to increased and more systematic toileting opportunities, or to the behavioural procedures. Nevertheless, despite these cases being identified as the worst cases of incontinence in non-bedfast clients, and despite a belief by nursing staff that a two-hour prompting schedule would not work, a substantial improvement was effected. These authors believe reinforcement of appropriate urination to be more effective than reinforcement of dry pants.

Using a reversal design, Spangler *et al.* (1984) compared standard nursing care with a one and half hourly prompted voiding and drinking procedure. No structured behavioural training procedures were used. In spite of increased fluid intake under the experimental procedure, eight residents became dry as opposed to two under standard nursing care. Schnelle *et al.* (1989) and Schnelle *et al.* (1990) report on a study of 126 severely cognitively and physically impaired nursing home residents aged between 65 and 99 years. Using a multiple baseline design, patients were checked at regular, set intervals, asked if they were wet or dry, given immediate feedback as to the correctness of the answer and praised if dry. Patients were then asked if they would like to visit the toilet. Treatment resulted in a significant decrease in incontinence and increase in appropriate toileting across the multiple baseline design. As with Pinkston *et al.* (1987), it is only possible to state that trainees responded to both increased toileting opportunities and rewards for continence. Colling *et al.* (1992) similarly found that urinary incontinence reduced in 51 physically and/or mentally impaired elderly nursing home residents compared to a control group upon implementation of a prompted voiding procedure, based on individual patterns of voiding, over a 12-week period. Reductions were more modest than those reported in other studies, though a change was nevertheless effected.

Hu *et al.* (1989) studied 143 women aged between 65 to 95 years, two thirds of whom were significantly cognitively impaired and few of whom were ambulant. Patients were randomly assigned to a 13 week behavioural treatment programme consisting of hourly checks and prompts to toilet, with praise and staff attention for appropriate urination and dryness at checks. Spontaneous toilet requests were encouraged and given social reinforcement. Training resulted in a significant reduction in incontinence over the control group though again less success was obtained than that found by Schnelle *et al.* (1989). Burgio *et al* (1988) studied four elderly incontinent but ambulant nursing home residents with cognitive impairment. A voiding programme was implemented with cognitive staff approval for dryness and appropriate toileting and corrective feedback for wetness. All four became substantially drier. Improvement was not related to age, mental status or toileting history.

As not all of these studies used additional training techniques from behavioural psychology, it is clear that some improvement can be effected simply by use of increased and more systematic toileting opportunities. However, where a structured behavioural approach is used, success is likely to be higher. There are many distinct components to a behaviourally based continence programme. As yet, however, no analysis has been carried out into the effectiveness of separate components, such as reinforcement of dry pants versus appropriate toilet use, with the elderly. It is useful, therefore, to draw parallels with other, related fields. Work on bladder training in mental handicap has shown that early studies focusing heavily on reinforcement of dry pants were unsuccessful, while later studies emphasising rewards for passing urine on the toilet were successful (see Smith and Smith, 1987 for discussion).

Failure to maintain changes

There is clear evidence from recent studies (Schnelle *et al.*, 1990; Burgio *et al.*, 1990) of the failure to change staff behaviour long term. Staff training, written instructions for maintaining continence gains and even success in training patient continence do not change staff attitudes and behaviour long term (Schnelle *et al.*, 1990). Schnelle *et al.* describe 91 nursing home residents with an average age of 82 years, 84% of whom could not toilet independently. When checked hourly, they were incontinent on about 30% of occasions. A programme to provide two-hourly toiletings reduced this incontinence rate to about 12% of occasions. However, follow up six weeks after staff training and monitoring had been completed showed reversal of incontinence rates to baseline levels. Burgio *et al.* (1990) had decreased incontinence and increased successful toiletings with a prompted voiding procedure for four elderly nursing home residents with dementia. However, four to five months after a self-monitoring and group feedback system was introduced, staff performance and patient success rate declined. When individual staff monitoring and feedback of performance were re-introduced, staff prompts to void and successful voidings increased once more. Colling *et al.* (1992) similarly found only a 70% staff compliance rate for prescribed toileting times for maintenance of continence gains. Goldstein *et al.* (1989) found that faecal continence, which had been successfully retrained in a 90 year old man living in the community, relapsed after his live in carer refused to carry out certain aspects required for maintenance of continence which she found distasteful. Campbell *et al.* (1991) found low compliance and staff resistance to change despite education, toileting protocols and continuing presence of project staff.

The obvious and important questions here focus on why and how staff are able to see improvements in continence in elderly people with dementia, yet do not necessarily change their own behaviour long term to maintain these improvements. Hu *et al.* (1989) suggest the existence of conflicting interests and needs among nursing home administrators, care staff and residents. They point out that nursing home objectives may be to minimise costs and maximise profits. Thus, to maintain continence, stressed care staff (usually unqualified) would have to increase their work output, and this is likely to conflict with their beliefs about the most efficient way to get the work done (Campbell *et al.*, 1991). Thomas *et al.* (1987), in their study of the prevalence and management of faecal incontinence in old people's homes in the UK, feel that staff morale in this area is not high. Miller (1984, 1985) has argued that the dependency of elderly patients is not solely determined by their physical or mental status but also by interaction effects between the patient and the environment, including rigid institutional nursing styles, with a considerable proportion of the measured dependency of 168 elderly patients arising from the type of nursing care they received.

The attitudes, beliefs and taboos associated with incontinence in the general population are reflected in the well documented reluctance of people to seek help from professionals for their incontinence (Thomas *et al.*, 1986; Norton *et al.*, 1988). Reasons include the belief that incontinence is 'normal' for old age and that 'nothing can be done anyway' (British Association of Continence Care, 1991; Simmons, 1985). Of concern also are professional knowledge and beliefs about the treatability of incontinence. Mitteness (1990) has recently reviewed some of the evidence in this field and the results are not encouraging. Among other problem professionals, too, frequently regard incontinence as intractable and normal in the elderly, so much so that measurable improvements in toileting behaviour in elderly people may not be perceived by their nurses (Tarrier and Larner, 1983).

Incontinence and dementia

One of the probable contributing factors to negative beliefs and attitudes about incontinence concerns professional beliefs about the nature of the links between dementia and incontinence. There are two possible ways in which incontinence and dementia might be associated; incontinence as a direct effect and incontinence as an indirect effect.

Arie *et al.* (1976) and Brocklehurst (1984) are among those who emphasise possible effects of specific lesions in dementia on urinary incontinence. No matter which type of dementia is involved, lesions at cortical or subcortical levels may very plausibly directly affect centres of bladder or bowel control. That the commonest form of urinary incontinence in dementia is said to be urge incontinence or detrusor instability may be interpreted as consistent with this view. The alternative view is that incontinence may be a secondary effect mediated by other factors such as confusion. A major cognitive feature of dementia is disorientation with respect to place and time, with additional factors such as short term memory and attentional deficits and the reduced effects of social consequences. Whitehead *et al.* (1984) have pointed out that if incontinence were due to a specific lesion, then one would expect the resulting incontinence to be total. The fact that the degree of incontinence tends to correlate with the severity of the dementia lends more support to the general association view and less to the specific lesion stance.

One intriguing recent study sheds some light on the relationship between cognitive impairment and incontinence (Davidson *et al.*, 1991). In this study, continence and incontinent patients with dementia were compared on the various subtests of the Mini Mental Status Exam. A striking association was found between incontinence and the inability to perform a cube copying task, with incontinent subjects scoring significantly lower. Analysis of the errors in the copying task revealed particularly poor representation of perspective and spatial orientation, features characteristic of rightsided parietal lesions. Thus, it is possible that localised cortical lesions are associated with one type of incontinence, but that the mechanisms is an indirect one through the mediation of spatial orientation. This is reminiscent of the study by Holden and Woods (1982), where a number of elderly women in a psychiatric hospital were rated as incontinent. Observation demonstrated that most of them could in fact successfully use the toilet once there, but had difficulty finding it.

Panella (1986) identifies four reasons for incontinence in patients with dementia, including inability to communiate needs, disorientation in space resulting in inability to locate toilet, disruption in sequencing resulting in confusion in the bathroom or a combination of the above. To this could probably be added social disinhibition and lack of motivation. Panella believes that patients with dementia are, however, aware of bladder and bowel function and therefore proposes three essential components to dealing with incontinence: physical plan and layout of bathroom, staff-related factors regarding toileting schedules, and the use of behavioural techniques. Many recent studies have successfully reduced incontinence rates in severely cognitively impaired people by concentrating on the second and third of these. Regular toileting schedules are both appropriate and effective. As dementia progresses, staff must prompt patients to the toilet verbally, then, as disorientation so space increases, must give verbal and physical prompts, then hands-on assistance for actual toileting, then total assistance (Panella, 1986).

The important point here concerns the implicit beliefs of care staff about the causes of faecal incontinence. If staff take a direct effect stance, then faecal incontinence will largely be viewed as intractable and irreversible. If staff accept that some incontinence may in fact be secondary to the dementia, then some of the environmental and training manipulations outlined in this chapter may be considered.

Staff training and management systems

Given a strong suggestion of indirect effects of dementia on continence, coupled with poor carer morale and the belief that incontinence is intractable, the question arises 'What can be done?'.

Thomas *et al.* (1987), in commenting on the problems of low morale, emphasise the importance of staff training. However, the experience of many across various long-stay residential settings such as mental illness, mental handicap and elderly, is that staff training alone rarely results in long term change in staff behaviour: Colling *et al.* (1992) failed to change staff knowledge and attitudes significantly through a four hour education programme, with nursing staff preferring to maintain current routines, probably party because toileting took longer to achieve than changing; and in Schnelle *et al.*'s (1990) study, staff were given training and written instructions for the maintenance of continence gains following a prompted voiding programme, but at follow up had failed to maintain the toileting schedules so that incontinence had regressed to the baseline level. In commenting that the additional time needed to maintain continence over and above that required to change an incontinent patient is the most plausible explanation for the failure to provide regular prompts to toilet, several authors conclude that better staff management procedures need to be devised to reverse habits that counter improvements in continence (Hu *et al.*, 1989; Schnelle *et al.*, 1990). Spangler *et al.* (1984) used regular data collection and performance checks by staff management to maintain gains after normal staff took over from project staff. Similarly, Burgio *et al.* (1988) and Engel *et al.* (1990) used individual staff monitoring and feedback and found this to be more effective than group feedback, while feedback plus contingencies in the form of 'official' letters 'always resulted in a significantly higher level of performance.'. Goldstein *et al.* (1989) propose a need for better support for carers, whether family or professional. This should include cognitive/behavioural therapy to help the carer find his or her role more satisfying, an educational component to provide better skills for coping with problem solving and anxiety management techniques to aid relaxation and reduce stress.

In institutional settings, where block treatment is often sadly the norm, it is clear that simplistic notions of providing either staff training or demonstration of improvements will not result in major long term changes. A more explicitly behavioural approach with use of incentives for change and maintenance of staff behaviour is indicated. Positive monitoring involving senior managers is also likely to be far more effective. Furthermore, the current move towards clearly establishing standards of care should involve measures of quality of life and patient dignity for the incontinent individual (Harke and Richgels, 1992).

It must be said that, having worked intensively in both large institutions and small community homes, attitudes to change tend to be more favourable in small community homes where living accommodation and staff patterns of behaviour are less subject to rigid routine and much more like normal family life. However, even in small community settings more akin to a normal living situation and where the principle of individual programmes for residents is more readily accepted, a high level of support and monitoring is nevertheless necessary. Biofeedback is a psychophysiological technique whereby abnormal physiological responses are measured and fed back to an individual so as to enable that individual to modify his responses towards normality, the assumption being that 'Underlying the behaviour is a psychophysiological system that maintains the symptoms of disorder' (Barowsky, 1990). Biofeedback has variously been applied to problems such as tension and headaches, irritable bowel, anxiety, diabetes and ashthma, using measures such as muscle tension, bowel sounds, heart rate, and blood glucose level. Biofeedback techniques are thus directed at unconditioned responses formerly thought to be outwith voluntary control (Engel, 1981). Biofeedback techniques have also been used in the treatment of incontinence of bowel and bladder.

A brief discussion of the assumptions underlying biofeedback treatment techniques is appropriate at this point, as biofeedback would appear on the face of it to be a fairly simple, rapid and inexpensive but effective technique. Yates (1985) provides a useful, critical but insightful discussion of the 'success' of biofeedback and the assumptions underlying its usage, to which the reader is referred. Assumptions underlying biofeedback have been accepted uncritically by clinical biofeedback therapists. Using as an example the problems of tension versus migraine headaches, Yates firstly demolishes the assumptions regarding the hypothesised respective and different underlying psychiological mechanisms for these, together with the biofeedback treatments which follow from the assumed mechanisms. He is equally dismissive of claims for the control of blood/glucose levels in diabetes through the use of biofeedback techniques, as well as of their use in the treatment of bronchial asthma or temperomandibular joint dysfunction. In all of these, the supposed relationships between the physiological measures and the disorder are unsupported by empirical evidence. In fact, according to yates, little correlation has been found between symptoms (e.g. heart rate, blood pressure, etc.) in any general way, though idiosyncratic patterns may exist for individuals. Latimer (1981) is similarly critical of biofeedback for the treatment of irritable bowel syndrome. Here, treatment has aimed to reduce bowel sounds on the assumption that these are a valid measure of bowel activity, increased bowel motility being a supposed characteristic of the syndrome. Studies are said to have produced conflicting results, have lacked proper controls and proper clinical outcome measures. Like Yates, Latimer agrees that what a person says, what he does and how he responds physiologically may not be highly correlated. Thus, change in bowel habit may be reported in the absence of any evidence of physiological abnormalities.

Where, then, does this leave us in relation to biofeedback training for faecal incontinence? Biofeedback is described variously as proven, without controversy and the treatment of choice for faecal incontinence (Constantinides and Cywes, 1983; MacLeod, 1987; Duckro *et al.*, 1985). It has been used for urinary and faecal incontinence in cases of CNS damage caused by mechanical injury such as childbirth or previous surgery, illness such as multiple sclerosis, congenital abnormality such as spina bifida, and accident such as head injury (Tries, 1990). Though Engel (1981) agrees that physiological responses like heart rate may not be a valid measure of behaviour or emotions such as anxiety, he nevertheless feels that physiological responses are valid in the understanding of behaviour where unconditioned responses are involved. He finds abnormalities in external and sphincter pressure, in threshold of rectal sensation and in coordination of internal and external sphincters. Biofeedback training therefore aims to reduce the threshold of sensation in the rectum, or increase the external sphincter response, or co-ordinate the action of internal and external sphincters, or all three.

The use of biofeedback to modify and sphincter responses was first described by Kohlenberg (1973) in a 13 year old boy, where inadequate and sphincter tone had been suggested to be the cause of encopresis. Anal sphincter responses were measured via a single balloon inserted in the rectum so as to cross the area of the anal sphincter. Whereas visual feedback with verbal instructions alone had little apparent effect on anal sphincter pressure, visual feedback in combination with operant reinforcement techniques increased anal sphincter pressures, which remained increased post-treatment. Unfortunately, though baseline measures of anal sphincter pressures were obtained, no objective base-line information is presented for the problem behaviour, namely soiling. Additionally, follow up at one year consisted solely of noting that neither the hospital nor the original referring physician had been re-contacted. Kohlenberg himself advises caution due to the 'causal nature of the . . . clinical reports and the unavailability of other follow-up data . . .'. Furthermore, any increase in resting anal sphincter pressure could have been due to increases in intra-abdominal pressure, a factor of which later workers tend to take account.

Using a three balloon system to measure rectal sensation as well as internal and external sphincter contraction, Engel *et al.* (1974) present information on six patients with severe faecal incontinence. Five out of six had no history of constipation or impaction but all were said to have diminished or absent external sphincter responses. Visual feedback plus verbal instructions as to the appearance of 'normal responses' were given in conjunction with praise for the production of a 'normal appearing' response. Though changes in physiological measures were objectively evaluated, assessment of the problem behaviour, i.e. incontinence, was again somewhat casual with no objective measures presented. However, four patients reported complete continence within four treatment sessions, with one experiencing 'rare' staining episodes. One patient required training to co-ordinate internal and external sphincter responses as well as for an absent external sphincter. All patients were said to demonstrate objective evidence of learned external sphincter control, though data is only presented for one individual and in polygraph form.

Cerulli *et al.* (1979) found incontinence to be cured or 90% decreased in 36 of 50 patients treated by the three balloon system. Causes of incontinence included previous anorectal surgery, irritable bowel syndrome, diabetes, rectal prolapse, multiple sclerosis, and stroke. Though the threshold for rectal sensation values were similar for good and poor responders before training, good responders decreased their threshold significantly more than poor responders with training. All patients had deficits in external sphincter function before training, which 'were corrected in the good response group'. No data is presented. No success was achieved for those with anal perforations.

Whitehead *et al.* (1985) studied 18 elderly people suffering from faecal incontinence and constipation, all of whom were able to walk at least a few steps. Six had both urinary and faecal incontinence. In addition, two suffered from dementia and three were depressed. Prior to the use of biofeedback, all patients were placed on a 'habit training' programme consisting of daily attempts to defaecate after breakfast, the use of enemas after two days without a bowel movement, and additional use of bulking agents in 11. Patients remaining incontinent after four weeks of habit training went on to biofeedback. Two patients with dementia were excluded together with one who could not perceive rectal distension. Two patients became continent on habit training and three were excluded as above. External anal sphincter contraction was significantly increased in the 13 biofeedback trainees, of whom six became continent and four achieved a 75% reduction in incontinence. At six month follow up, five of these ten were continent or only had rare soilings. Those treated with habit training only 'continued to improve'. An average of 4.1 biofeedback sessions was required. No factors are presented to account for poor clinical response to biofeedback in the three who were clinical failures despite their 'significantly increased' anal sphincter contractions. These should presumably have critically remained unchanged. No data is presented for the six month follow up for those cases who relapsed. Measures of urinary incontinence for those additionally incontinent of urine would be of interest, as urinary incontinence should critically remain unchanged while faecal incontinence improved.

Of interest to us is Whitehead *et al.*'s exclusion of two patients suffering from dementia and their conclusion that other behavioural approaches would be more appropriate. Providing the elderly person with dementia is not generally agitated or distressed, cognitive impairment in itself need not be a reason for exclusion, though treatment is likely to be prolonged. Although the principle of feedback would remain the same, the actual techniques of providing feedback may be qualitatively different. Thus, praise and other more concrete methods of reinforcement appropriate to the individual would be combined with a more highly structured, behavioural shaping approach such as that used by McCubbin *et al.* (1987).

Duckro *et al.* (1985) report on the use of biofeedback and behavioural therapy training in a seven year old boy with uretersigmoidostomy and subsequent anal soiling of liquid stool. Psychiatric intervention had been recommended, initiated and had failed to improve the situation. In this case, biofeedback used surface EMG feedback of perianal muscles, which the patient was taught to contract while relaxing the lower abdomen. Rewards were used for continence but the maintenance of patient motivation was problematic Incontinence was considerably reduced though not eliminated. The most crucial point made by the authors relates to the difficulty of ascertaining the exact role of the biofeedback training, as there was 'no real progression in the perianal EMG'. In fact, at one stage, an actual decrease in EMG performance occurred but with no corresponding increase in incontinence. Training effects could therefore have been due to the behavioural intervention and not the biofeedback.

Sims *et al.* (1987) present the case of one 46 year old woman with paraplegia due to multiple sclerosis, who was suffering from 'chronic faecal retention and occasional incontinence'. Training was reported to have resulted in a substantial reduction in amount of time spent on the toilet before initiating a bowel movement. Data is not reported for retention and incontinence. Furthermore, no data is given to indicate whether or not corresponding EMG changes occurred.

McCubbin *et al.* (1987) report on the successful treatment of chronic constipation without incontinence in an adult female, where sphincter reflexes were normal but threshold for rectal sensation was abnormally elevated. Biofeedback sensory discrimination training resulted in a greater frequency of bowel movements and decreased use of laxatives. This study used a highly behaviourally based shaping procedure to train the desired response by starting at the volume of air which could be successfully detected on 50% of occasions and training at this level until 70% successful response had been achieved, before moving to the next level. Few biofeedback studies have approached training in this way, with starting points for training and criteria for moving on usually being somewhat haphazard.

MacLeod (1987) reports on a study of 113 patients using training of the external sphincter only, where standard pelvic floor exercises had previously failed to achieve improvement. Sixty three percent of patients either became continent or had at least a 90% reduction in incontinence in three to four sessions, with no relapses at follow up of minimum six months. Interestingly, hospital treated patients did worse than office based patients, a fact which MacLeod attributes to the hospital based treatment being carried out by technicians, albeit highly trained. The procedure was found to be most successful for post-obstetric or post-surgery incontinence, radiation induced or idiopathic incontinence, and less successful for neurological causes and rectal prolapse and, like Cerulli, not successful at all with anal perforations. MacLeod asserts that internal sphincter relaxation and rectal sensation are not critical factors, as his successes were achieved through external sphincter training alone. However, the fact that 56 of his patients were said to have had no sensory deficit implies that 57 did, but that gains in continence with these patients were achieved without sensory training, which in theory they should have required. Additionally, MacLeod reports that several patients became continent with no measured improvement in external sphincter performance! He views this contradiction as a function of issues surrounding different types of biofeedback equipment, rather than the sort of very basic theoretical issues raised by Yates and Latimer.

Burton *et al.* (1988) compared six biofeedback sessions and six 'behavioural training' sessions for urinary incontinence in 28 patients aged 64–83 years. Patients were cognitively intact, did not have functional or overflow incontinence (though cystometry was not carried out), major psychiatric disorders or physical disability. Behavioural training consisted of an explanation of the mechanisms of bowel and bladder control and explanations to help achieve continence, e.g. by stop-start exercises for stress incontinence; or relaxing and tightening the urethral sphincter while relaxing the abdominal muscles, then going slowly to lavatory to void for urge incontinence. Both groups achieved a comparable reduction in urinary accidents: 79% for biofeedback and 82% for behavioural training. Follow-up showed gains maintained at six months. No control group was used though the authors appear to feel there is no real need for this in the case of longstanding incontinence and where a two week baseline period is used. These results, according to the authors, are only applicable to cognitively intact, ambulant, independent and motivated patients. As 'behavioural training' is a term loosely used here for techniques which most psychologists would regard rather as counselling, results for the biofeedback training are thus not impressive.

Leoning-Baucke *et al.* (1988) are critical of many of the biofeedback studies for their failure to use a control group. Twelve children with faecal incontinence due to myelomeningocoele, a group with whom Cerulli *et al.* (1979) obtained a poorer response, and 16 controls were studied. Four of the treatment group were then assigned to a 'habit training' group and eight to this plus three biofeedback sessions. Biofeedback training used a combination of the three balloon system in the clinic setting and an anal canal balloon for home training. Six month evaluation found no significant difference in soiling frequency between habit training and biofeedback groups. Three out of four habit trained and three out of eight biofeedback trained showed a good response. Measures such as anal sphincter response and threshold of rectal sensation, among many others, were not significantly different after treatment between groups, or from pre- to post-treatment within groups. Nor were any of these measures significantly different for those with good versus poor outcome. The authors are critical of studies which have found differences in external and response after treatment, believing this to be an artifact of the positioning of the external balloon. Like many biofeedback studies, the behavioural measures used in this study were less satisfactory, with diaries used for baseline but a questionnaire on incontinence for follow up.

Loening-Baucke (1990) compared anorectal measures for two groups of faecally incontinent women treated either with medical treatment alone to improve stool consistency, or medical treatment plus bio-feedback training using the three balloon system. Patients whose incontinence was caused by conditions known to have a poor prognosis in terms of treatment had been excluded. Neither soiling frequency nor anorectal measures were found to differ significantly between the groups after treatment, either immediately or at one year follow up.

Latimer *et al.* (1984) carried out a components analysis of biofeedback in the treatment of faecal incontinence. Biofeedback for faecal incon-tinence is, according to these authors, one of the few applications of this techniue which appears to be clinically effective, yet no controlled studies or component analyses have been carried out. In a study of eight patients aged between eight and 72 years, and using a randomised trial of external sphincter exercise training, sensory discrimination training and full biofeedback training for each patient, they, like other authors, found biofeedback to be an effective and rapid treatment for faecal incontinence. Major accidents were reduced for seven of the eight patients. However, only one of the eight required the full biofeedback training; three responded to sensory discrimination training alone; one with normal sensation responded to exercise training alone; one did not maintain response to any aspect of biofeedback until other behavioural methods were implemented; and at least one, arguably two, got better with no treatment at all. However, of greatest theoretical interest, using the baseline manometric data to predict outcome, four patients would have been predicted to respond to sensory discrimination training and did; in three who would have been predicted to require exercise training, one failed to respond to this and two responded instead to discrimination training which happened to come first but which they should not have required; of three patients who had no measurable deficits at all but who were nevertheless incontinent, one or two got better with no treatment and one required contingency management.

Finally, Miner *et al.* (1990) studied a group of faecally incontinent patients initially allocated either to active (feedback) or sham (no feed-back) sensory retraining groups. Sham sensory retraining was followed by active retraining, with all patients subsequently receiving training for external sphincter strength as well as training to co-ordinate internal and external sphincters, in a cross-over design. Frequency of incontinent episodes was reduced in both 'feedback' and 'no feedback' groups but, though the magnitude of improvement was greater for the feedback group with four patients becoming fully continent compared to none in the control group, these differences were not significant. Small sample sizes might, of course, account for these differences failing to reach statistical significance. Although the authors conclude that '. . . it is gratifying that a relatively brief period of retraining can improve faecal continence in many patients . . .', they admit that the physiological basis for this remains, nevertheless, unclear and that they '. . . could not demonstrate that this improvement was associated with any significant change in any of the objective indices of sphincter function'.

To conclude, although biofeedback training seems to be a relatively quick, simple and inexpensive method of training faecal continence, closer inspection reveals major, as yet unanswered questions relating to the precise relationship between continence, incontinence and various physiological measures of bowel function (Miner *et al.*, 1990; Loening-Baucke, 1990). There is evidence that people do not become continent despite showing physiological changes, while others become continent with no physiological changes; that some become continent after bio-feedback training of responses which they should not have required training in; and that some become continent before training begins. The situation is by no means clear as it might have initially appeared. Though the procedure might appear simple to clinicians, the appearance of the biofeedback equipment and the procedures involved in their use might be sufficiently impressive to result in a substantial placebo effect. At any rate, a clear superiority of biofeedback training over habit training, counselling or more structured behavioural techniques has not yet been demonstrated. The difficulty in comparing the above studies is that they use different types of equipment, measure physiological responses at different sites, for subjects with different diagnoses and different ages. Sample sizes are small, behavioural measures and follow up data are usually poor, data is presented in different ways, with anorectal measures before and after training often not presented at all. Although biofeedback results are promising, it is clear that much work remains to be carried out.

Other psychological approaches: anxiety reduction

Paradoxical instruction or paradoxical intention is used where a problem is assumed to have a substantial component of performance related anxiety (Bornstein *et al.*, 1981; Propp, 1986). Here, the assumption is that toileting and related activities cause considerable anxiety. The harder a client tries to perform, perhaps because of the fear of incontinence or the fear of being unable to perform, the more anxiety is raised and the less likely he is to succeed. Bornstein describes the technique as follows: 'Paradoxical instruction techniques direct and encourage the client in the continuation of their problem behaviour with the paradoxical intent of symptomatic relief'. The patient is instructed *not* to perform the behaviour in question. Thus, the patient has to go to the toilet every hour, pull the pants down, sit for five minutes, act as if he has to do a bowel movement, but *should not allow that to occur*. using an ABAB reversal design, Bornstein demonstrated a clear effect. Treatment was brief and maintenance successful at one year.

The main advantage of this technique is that all aversive consequences such as may be involved in other behavioural techniques can be avoided. The obvious disadvantage is that it relies on ability to comprehend instructions and hence on largely intact cognitive abilities which may not be available in the mentally handicapped or elderly mentally infirm. Stoylen (1988) refers to a case of chronic constipation and defaecation rituals. Anxiety about constipation and failure to perform resulted in obsessional 'checking' trips in an attempt to perform. These trips began to assume an increasingly obsessional, ritualistic appearance when the client found he had to sit on a particular toilet and perform particular sets of movements in order to start the evacuation response. Treatment was successfully carried out using a standard technique of response prevention for obsessive compulsive behaviours except for permitted trips to toilet at specified times of the day. Similar types of behaviour problems have been noted and successfully treated in elderly people making constant demands for trips to toilet with a high false negative rate (Tarrier and Larner, 1983).

References

Arie T, Clarke M, Slattery Z. (1976) Incontinence in geriatric psychiatry. In: Willington FL (ed) *Incontinence in the Elderly*. Academic Press, New York.

Ayllon T, Simm SJ, Wildman RW. (1975) Instructions and reinforcements in the elimination of encopresis: a case study. *J Behav Ther Exp Psychiat*; **6**: 235–8.

Bach R, Moylan JJ. (1975) Parents administer behaviour therapy for inappropriate urination and encopresis: a case study. *J Behav Ther Exp Psychiat*; **6**: 239–41.

Balson J, Gartley CB, Humpal JJ. (1985) Personal experiences – people managing incontinence. In: Gartley CB (ed) *Managing Incontinence – A Guide to Living with Loss of Bladder Control*. Jameson Books, Illinois.

Barowsky E. (1990) The use of biofeedback in the treatment of disorders of childhood. *Ann N Y Acad Sci*; **602**: 221–3.

Berg I, Forsythe I, Holt P, Watts J. (1983) A controlled trial of 'Senokot' in faecal soiling treated by behavioural methods. *J Child Psychol Psychiat*; **24**: 543–9.

Berrigan LP, Stedman JM. (1989) Combined application of behavioural techniques and family therapy for the treatment of childhood encopresis: a strategic approach. *Fam Ther*; **16**: 51–7.

Blackwell C. (1990) The acquisition of noctural dryness in a population of 2–3 and 3–4 year old children. Unpublished MSc thesis in clinical psychology, University of Newcastle upon Tyne.

Bollard T, Nettlebeck J. (1982) A components analysis of dry bed training for childhood bedwetting. *Behav Res Ther*; **20**: 383–90.

Bornstein PH, Sturm CA, Retzlaff PD, Kirby KL, Chong H. (1981) Paradoxical instruction in the treatment of encopresis and chronic constipation: an experimental analysis. *J Behav Ther Exp Psychiat*; **12**: 167–70.

Bornstein PH, Balleweg BJ, McClellarn RW, et al. The 'bathroom game': a systematic program for the elimination of encopretic behavior. *J Behav Ther Exp Psychiat*; **14**: 67–71.

Borthwick J. (1985) Incontinence. Speaking from experience. *Nursing Times*; 3 April.

Bosch JD. (1988) Treating children with encopresis and constipation: an evaluation by means of single case studies. In: Emmelkamp P, Everaerd W, Kraaimat FR, Van Son MJM (eds) *Advances in Theory and Practice in Behaviour Therapy.* Swets and Zeitllinger, Amsterdam.

British Association of Continence Care. (1991) Mori 1990 Poll, Health Survey Questionaire.

Brocklehurst JC. (1984) Ageing, bladder function and incontinence. In: Brocklehurst JC (ed) *Urology in the Elderly.* Churchill Livingston, Edinburgh.

Brown B, Doolan M. (1983) Behavioural treatment of faecal soiling: a case study. *Behav Psychother;* **11**: 18–24.

Bulkeley R, Sahami V. (1983) Treatment of longstanding encopresis in a 12 year old boy using behaviour modification within a framework of systems theory. *Fam Ther;* **10**: 23–6.

Burgio LD, Engel BT, Hawkins A, McCormick K, Scheve A, Jones LT. (1990). A staff management system for maintaining improvements in continence with elderly nursing home residents. *J Appl Behav Anal;* **31**: 111–18.

Burgio L, Engel BT, McCormick K, Hawkins A, Scheve A. (1988) Behavioral treatment for urinary incontinence in elderly in-patients: initial attempts to modify prompting and toileting procedures. *Behav Ther;* **19**: 345–57.

Burton JR, Pearce KL, Burgio KL, Engel BT, Whitehead WE. (1988) Behavioral training for urinary incontinence in elderly ambulatory patients. *J Am Geriat Soc ;* **36**: 693–8.

Campbell EB, Knight M, Benson M, Colling J. (1991) Effect of an incontinence training program on nursing home staff's knowledge, attitudes and behaviour. *Gerontologist;* **31**: 788–94.

Cerulli MA, Nikoomanesh P, Schuster MM. (1979) Progress in biofeedback conditioning for faecal incontinence. *Gastroenterology;* **76**: 742–6.

Colling J, Ouslander J, Hadley B, Eisch J, Campbell E. (1992) The effect of patterned urge-response toileting (PURT) on urinary incontinence among nursing home residents. *J Am Geriat Soc;* **40**: 135–41.

Constantinides C, Cywes S. (1983). Faecal incontinence: a simple pneumatic device for home biofeedback training. *J Pediat Surg;* **18**: 276–7.

Davidson HA, Borrie MJ, Crilly RG. (1991) Copy task performance and urinary incontinence in Alzheimer's disease. *J Am Geriat Soc;* **39**: 467–71.

Davis HM, Mitchell WS, Marks FM. (1976) A behavioural programme for the modification of encopresis. *Child: Care, Health Develop;* **2**: 273–82.

Davis HM, Mitchell WS, Marks FM. (1977) A pilot study of encopretic children treated by behaviour modification. *Practitioner;* **219**: 228–30.

Dawson PM, Griffith K, Boeke KM. (1990) Combined medical and psychological treatment of hospitalised children with encopresis. *Child Psychiat Human Devel* **20**: 181–90.

Doleys DM. (1978) Assessment and treatment of enuresis and encopresis in children. In: Hersen M, Eisler R, Miller P (eds) *Progress in Behavior Modification (Vol. 6).* Academic Press, New York.

Doleys DM, Schwartz MS, Ciminero AR. (1981). Elimination problems: enuresis and encopresis. In: Mash EJ, Terdal LG (eds) *Behavioral Assessment of Childhood Disorders.* Guilford Press, New York.

Donald I, Smith R, Cruikshank J, Elton R, Stoddart M. (1985) A study of constipation in the elderly living at home. *Gerontology;* **31**: 112–18.

Drossman DA, Sandler RS, Broom CM, McKee DC. (1986) Urgency and faecal soiling in people with bowel dysfunction. *Dig Dis Sci;* **31**: 1221–5.

Duckro PN, Purcell M, Gregory J, Schultz K. (1985) Biofeedback for the treatment of anal incontinence in a child with utersigmoidostomy. *Biofeedback Self-Regulation;* **10**: 325–33.

Duker PC. (1983) Determinants of diurnal bladder control with institutionalised mentally retarded individuals. *Am J Mental Def;* **87**: 606–10.

Ehrmann JS. (1983) Use of biofeedback to treat incontinence. *J Am Geriat Soc*; **31**: 182–4.

Engel BT. (1981) Clinical biofeedback: a behavioral analysis. *Neurosci Behav Rev*; **5**: 397–400.

Engel BT, Burgio LD, McCormick KA, Hawkins A, Scheve A, Leahy E. (1990) Behavioral treatment of incontinence in the long-term care setting. *J Am Geriat Soc*; **38**: 361–3.

Engel BT. (1981) Clinical biofeedback: a behavioral analysis. *Neurosci Behav Rev*; **5**: 397–400.

Fischer M, Adkins W, Hall L, Scaman P, Hsi S, Marlett J. (1985) The effects of dietary fibre in a liquid diet on bowel function of mentally retarded individuals. *J Mental Def Res*; **29**: 373–81.

Foxx RM. (1985) The successful treatment of diurnal and nocturnal enuresis and encopresis. *Child Fam Behav Ther*; **17**: 39–47.

Friman PC, Mathews JR, Finney JW, Christopherson ER, Leibowitz JM. (1988) Do encopretic children have clinical significant behavior problems? *Pediatrics*; **2**: 407–9.

Gabel S, Hegedus AM, Wald A, Chandra R, Chiponis D. (1986) Prevalence of behavior problems and mental health utilization among encopretic children: implications for behavioral pediatrics. *Devel Behav Pediat*; **7**: 293–7.

Gartley CB, Humpal JJ. (1984) Individual socio-psychological coping mechanisms of the incontinent. Proceedings of the 14th Annual Meeting of the International Continence Society, Innsbruck, September, 355–6.

Goldstein MK, Brown EM, Holt P, Gallagher D, Winograd CH. (1989) Faecal incontinence in an elderly man. *J Am Geriat Soc*; **37**: 991–1002.

Harke JM, Richgels K. (1992) Barriers to implementing a continence programme in nursing homes. Unpublished paper, School of Nursing, University of Wisconsin, Madison.

Heaton KW. (1990) Dietary fibre. *Br Med J*; **300**: 1479–80.

Hereford SM, Clelland SC, Fellner M. (1973) Territoriality and scent marking. *m J Mental Def*; **77**: 426–30.

Herzog AR, Fultz NH, Brock BM, Brown MB, Diokno AC. (1988) Urinary incontinence and psychological distress among older adults. *Age and Ageing*; **3**: 115–21.

Holden UP, Woods RT. (1982) *Reality Orientation: Psychological Approaches to the Confused Elderly*. Churchill Livingstone, Edinburgh.

Houts AC, Mellon MW, Whelan JP. (1988) Use of dietary fibre and stimulus control to treat retentive encopresis: a multiple baseline investigation. *J Pediat Psychol*; **13**: 435–45.

Houts AC, Peterson JK. (1986) Treatment of a retentive encopretic child using contingency management and dietary modification with stimulus control. *J Pediat Psychol*; **11**: 375–83.

Hu T-W, Igou JF, Kaltreider DL, *et al.* (1989) A clinical trial of a behavioral therapy to reduce urinary incontinence in nursing homes. *J Am Med Assoc*; **261**: 2656–62.

Jeter KF, Wagner DB. (1990) Incontinence in the American home. *J Am Geriat Soc*; **38**: 379–83.

Kaplan BJ. (1985) A clinical demonstration program of a psychobiological application to childhood encopresis. *J Child Care*; **2**: 47–54.

Kira A. (1976) *The Bathroom* (2nd ed). Penguin Books. Harmondsworth.

Knell SM, Moore DJ. (1990) Cognitive-behavior play therapy in the treatment of encopresis. *J Clin Child Psychol*; **19**: 55–60.

Knell SM, Moore DJ. (1990) Cognitive-behavior play therapy in the treatment of encopresis. *J Clin Child Psychol*; **19**: 55–60.

Kohlenberg RJ. (1973) Operant conditioning of human anal sphincter pressure. *J Appl Behav Anal*; **6**: 201–8.

Kolko DJ. (1989) In-patient intervention for chronic functional encopresis in psychiatrically disturbed children. *Behav Res Treatment*; **4**: 231–52.

Landman GB, Levine MD, Rappaport L. (1983) A study of treatment resistance among children referred for encopresis. *Clin Pediat*; **23**: 449–52.

Landman GB, Rappaport L, Fenton T, Levine MD. (1986) Locus of control and self-esteem in children with encopresis. *Devel Behav Pediat*; **7**: 111–13.

Latimer P. (1981) Biofeedback and behavior disorders of the gastrointestinal tract. *Psychother Psychosom*; **36**: 200–12.

Latimer P, Campbell D, Kasperski J. (1984) A components analysis of biofeedback in the treatment of faecal incontinence. *Biofeedback Self-Regulation*; **19**: 311–24.

Levine MD, Bakow H. (1976) Children with encopresis: a study of treatment outcome. *Pediatrics*; **58**: 845–52.

Liebl B, Fischer M, van Calcar S, Marlett J. (1990) Dietary fiber and long-term large bowel response in enterally nourished nonambulatory profoundly retarded youth. *J Parent Ent Nut*; **14**: 371–5.

Loening-Baucke V. (1984a) Sensitivity of sigmoid colon and rectum in children treated for chronic constipation. *J Pediat Gastroenterol Nut*; **3**: 454–9.

Loening-Baucke V. (1984b) Abnormal rectoanal function in children recovered from chronic constipation and encopresis. *Gastroenterology*; **87**: 1299–1304.

Loening-Baucke V, Desch L, Wolraich M. (1988) Biofeedback training for patients with myelomeningocele and faecal incontinence. *Dev Med Child Neurol*; **30**: 781–90.

Loening-Baucke V. (1990) Efficacy of biofeedback training in improving faecal incontinence and anorectal physiologic function. *Gut*; **31**: 1395–1402.

Lupson S, Walton D. (1981) A trial of bran to relieve constipation in young mentally and physically handicapped patients. *Apex*; **9**: 64–6.

Lyon MA. (1984) Positive reinforcement and logical consequences in the treatment of classroom encopresis. *School Psychol Rev*; **13**: 238–43.

Macauley AJ, Stern RS, Holmes DM, Stanton SL. (1987) Micturition and the mind: psychological factors in the aetiology and treatment of urinary symptoms in women. *Br Med J*; **294**: 540–3.

MacLeod J. (1987) Management of anal incontinence by biofeedback. *Gastroenterology*; **93**: 291–4.

Masham, Baroness. (1985) Continence. Speaking from experience – keeping to routine. *Nursing Times*; 3 April.

McCubbin J, Surwit R, Mansbach C. (1987) Sensory discrimination training in the treatment of a case of chronic constipation. *Behav Ther*; **18**: 273–8.

Miller A. (1984) Nurse/patient dependency – a review of different approaches with particular reference to studies of the dependency of elderly patients. *J Adv Nurs*; **9**: 479–86.

Miller A. (1985) Nurse/patient dependency – is it iatrogenic? *J Adv Nurs*; **9** 479–86.

Miner PB, Donnelly TC, Read NW. (1990) Investigations of mode of action of biofeedback in treatment of faecal incontinence *Dig Dis Sci*; **35**: 1291–8.

Mitteness LS. (1990) Knowledge and beliefs about urinary incontinence in adulthood and old age. *J Am Geriat Soc*; **38**: 374–8.

Noelker LS. (1987) Incontinence in the elderly cared for by family. *Gerontologist*; **27**: 194–200.

Norton KRW, Bhat AV, Stanton SL. (1990) Psychiatric aspects of urinary incontinence in women attending an out-patient urodynamic clinic. *Br Med J*; **301**: 271–2.

Norton PA, MacDonald LD, Sedgewick PM, Stanton SL. (1988) Distress and delay associated with urinary incontinence, frequency and urgency in women. *Br Med J* **297**: 1187–9.

O'Brien S, Ross LV, Christopherson ER. (1986) Primary encopresis: evaluation and treatment. *J Appl Behav Anal*; **19**: 137–45.

Ouslander JG, Abelson F. (1990) Perceptions of urinary incontinence among elderly out-patients. *Gerontologist*; **30**: 369–72.

Owens-Stively J. (1987) Self-esteem and compliance in encopretic children. *Child Psychiat Human Devel*; **18**: 13–21.

Palmer MH. (1988) Incontinence: the magnitude of the problem. *Nurs Clin N Am*; **23**: 139–57.

Panella J. (1986) Toileting strategies in day care programs for dementia. *Clin Gerontol*; **4**: 61–3.

Pfadt A, Sullivan K. (1980) Application and data based modification of overcorrection training in an institutional toilet training program. Paper presented at the Association for the Advancement of Behavior Therapy, 14th Annual Conference, New York, November.

Pinkston EM, Howe MW, Blackman DK. (1987) Medical social work management of urinary incontinence in the elderly: a behavioral approach. *J Soc Serv Res*; **10**: 179–94.

Plachetta KM. (1976) Encopresis: a case study utilizing contracting, scheduling and self-charting. *J Behav Ther Exp Psychiat*; **7**: 195–6.

Propp L. (1986) A self-control treatment for encopresis combining self-charting with paradoxical instructions: two case examples. *J Child Adol Psychother*; **2**: 26–31.

Resnick B. (1985) Constipation: common but preventable. *Geriat Nurs*; July/August, 213–15.

Rolider A, van Houten R. (1985) Treatment of constipation caused encopresis by a negative reinforcement procedure. *J Behav Ther Exp Psychiat*; **16**: 67–70.

Rosenthal MJ, Marshall CE. (1987) Sigmoid volvolus in association with parkinsonian: report of four cases. *J Geriat Soc*; **35**: 683–4.

Rovetto F. (1979) Treatment of chronic constipation by classical conditioning techniques. *J Behav Ther Exp Psychiat*; **10**: 143–6.

Sabin N. (1990) An examination of the prevalence and determina of urinary and faecal incontinence. In: Patient psychiatric population. Unpublished Msc Dissertation, Dept. of Clinical Psychology, University of Newcastle upon Tyne.

Sanavio E. (1981) Toilet retaining of psychogeriatric residents. *Behav Mod*; : 417–27.

Sandler RS, Drossman DA, Nathan HP, McKee DC. (1985) Symptom complaints and health care seeking behaviour in subjects with bowel dysfunction. *Gastroenterology*; **87**: 314–18.

Schaeffer CE. (1979) *Childhood Enuresis and Encopresis: Causes and Therapy*. van Nostrand Reinhold, New York.

Schenelle JF, Newman DR, Fogarty T. (1990) Management of patient continence in long-term care nursing facilities. *Gerontologist*; **30**: 373–6.

Schnelle JF, Traughber B, Sowell VA, Newman DR, Petrilli CO, Ory M. (1989) Prompted voiding treatment of urinary incontinence in nursing home patients. *J Am Geriat Soc*; **37**: 1051–7.

Shrubsole L, Smith PS. (1984) The effect of change in environment on incontinence in profoundly mentally handicapped adults. *Br J Mental Subnormality*; **30**: 44–53.

Simons J. (1985) Does incontinence affect your client's self-concept? *J Gerontol Nurs*; **11**: 37–40.

Sims CG, Remler H, Cox CD. (1987) Biofeedback and behavioral treatment of elimination disorders. *Clin Biofeedback Health*; **10**: 115–22.

Smith PS. (1979) The development of urinary continence in the mentally handicapped. Unpublished PhD thesis in clinical psychology, University of Newcastle upon Tyne.

Smith PS, Smith LJ. (1987) *Continence and incontinence: psychological approaches to development and treatment.* Croom Helm, London.

Spangler PF, Risley TR, Bilyew DD. (1984) The management of dehydration and incontinence in nonambulatory geriatric patients. *J Appl Behav Anal*; **17**: 397–401.

Sroujieh AS. (1988) Phytobezoars of the whole gastro-intestinal tract: report of a case and review of the literature. *Dirasat*; **15**: 103–9.

Stark LJ, Spirito A, Lewis AV, Hart KJ. (1990) Encopresis: behavioral parameters associated with children who fail medical management. *Child Psychiat Human Devel*; **20**: 169–79.

Steege MW, Harper DC. (1989) Enhancing the management of secondary encopresis by assessing acceptability of treatment: a case study. *J Behav Ther Exp Psychiat*; **20**: 333–41.

Stoylen IJ. (1988) Psychogenic defecation rituals with constipation – a case study. *Scand J Behav Ther*; **17**: 231–8.

Tarrier N, Larner S. (1983) The effects of manipulation of social reinforcement on toilet requests on a geriatric ward. *Age and Ageing*; **12**: 234–9.

Thomas TM. (1986) The prevalence and health service implications of incontinence – a study in progress. In: Mandelstam D (ed) *Incontinence and Its Management* (2nd ed). Croom Helm, London.

Thomas TM, Ruff C, Karran O, Mellows S, Meade TW. (1987) A study of the prevalence and management of patients with faecal incontinence on old people's homes. *Comm Med*; **9**: 232–7.

Thompson WG, Heaton KW. (1980) Functional bowel disorders in apparently healthy people. *Gastroenterology*; **79**: 27–30.

Tries J. (1990) The use of biofeedback in the treatment of incontinence due to head injury. *J Head Trauma Rehab*; **5**: 91–100.

Turner RK, Corp M, Rousseau E, Heeraman P. (1986) Mental Health Services Unit continence survey. Unpublished Report. Towers Hospital, Leicestershire Health Authority.

Vidailhet C. (1983) Clinical study. *Neuropsychiatrie de l'Enfance et de l'Adolescence*; **31**: 197–200.

Webster A, Gore E. (1980) The treatment of intractable encopresis: a team intervention approach. *Child: Care, Health Devel*; **6**: 351–60.

Whitehead WE, Burgio KL, Engel BT. (1984) Behavioral methods in the assessment and treatment of urinary incontinence. In: Brocklehurst JC (ed) *Urology in the Elderly*. Churchill Livingstone, Edinburgh.

Whitehead We, Burgio KL, Engel BT. (1985) Biofeedback of faecal incontinence in geriatric patients. *J Am Geriat Soc*; **33**: 320–4.

Whitehead WE, Drinkwater D, Cheskin L, Heller B, Schuster M. (1989) Constipation in the elderly living at home. *J Am Geriat Soc*; **37**: 423–9.

Wyman JF, Harkins SW, Choi SC, Taylor JR, Fantl JA. (1987) Psychosocial impact of urinary incontinence in women. *Obstet Gynecol*; **70**: 378–81.

Syman JF, Harkins SW, Fantl JA. (1990) Psychosocial impact of urinary incontinence in the community-dwelling population. *J Am Geriat Soc*; **38**: 282–8.

Yates AJ. (1985) The relevance of fundamental research to clinical applications of biofeedback. In: Reiss S, Bootzin RR (eds) *Theoretical Issues in Behavior Therapy*. Academic Press, New York.

Yu LC. (1987) Incontinence stress index; measuring psychosocial impact. *J Gerontol Nurs*; **13**: 18–25.

Yu LC, Kaltreider DL. (1987) Stressed nurses dealing with incontinent patients. *J Gerontol Nurs*; **13**: 27–30.

Index

Abdominal massage in treatment   139
Acetylcholine
  effect on sphincter muscle   8
Acquired immunodeficiency
    syndrome
  diarrhoea in   151
Activity
  gut transit and   30
Ageing
  anal resting pressure and   61
  anal sensation and   67, 74, 112
  anorectal angle and   67
  anorectal function and   60–75
  anorectal incontinence and   47
  bowel habits and   60
  colonic motility and   61
  Crohn's disease and   82
  defaecation and   67
  denervation and   62, 63
  effect on anal squeeze pressure   61
  external sphincter and   61, 71
  nerve conduction changes in   64
  orocaecal transit time and   90
  pudendal nerve terminal motor
    latency and   64
  rectal sensation and   65
  recto-anal reflex and   65
  ulcerative colitis and   81
Alzheimer's disease   114, 122
  see also Dementia
Anal canal
  activity of   20
  anatomy of   5
  flutter valve action   25
  short   163
  slit-shaped   25
Anal canal pressure
  during micturition   20
  hourly variations in   23
  intra-abdominal pressure
    affecting   21
Anal canal sensation
  ageing and   112
Anal cushions in continence   25
Anal dilation
  sphincter injury following   40
Anal endosonography   40
Anal function
  assessment of   12–7
  electromyography   15
  manometric studies   12
  microtransducer recording
    devices   14
  recto-anal inhibitory reflex   14
  strain gauge systems for   13
Anal manometry   12, 110

Anal pain after therapy   161
Anal plugs   171, 172
Anal pressure   22
  see also Anal resting pressure and Anal
    squeeze pressure
  anal cushions and   26
  anal sensation and   48
  assessment of   131
  biofeedback and   158
  continence and   22
  hypertrophied anal cushions
    and   26
  inflation reflex   21
  sex differences in   19
  variation in   23
Anal reflex
  in anorectal incontinence   42
Anal resting pressure   6
  after electrical stimulation   160
  after postanal repair   162
  biofeedback and   158
  in continence   46
  defaecation and   118
  in dementia   118
  in descending perineum
    syndrome   49
  effect of age on   61
  estimation of   131
  in faecal impaction   72, 110
  in faecal loading   72, 127
  in incontinence   46, 125
  internal sphincter thickness
    and   49
  measurement   13
  mobility and   66
  in multiple sclerosis   53
  normal   13
  obstetric factors   45
  position and   20
  in prolapse   47, 49
  sphincter pressure and   51
  in spinal cord lesions   55
Anal sensation   8
  age affecting   67, 74, 112
  in anorectal incontinence   47
  continence and   48
  in faecal incontinence   74
  loss of   74
  obstetric factors   45
  pressures and   48
  temperature and   23
Anal sphincters
  artificial   164
  biofeedback modifying   195
  denervation of   64
  dilation causing injury   40

diurnal variation in   20
effect of rectal distension on   21
endosonography of   40
injury to   40
nerve supply to   6
obstetric damage to   43, 44, 45
pressure in diabetes   52
role in continence   118
squeeze and resting pressures
   and   119
Anal sphincter, external
   activity of   18
   ageing and   61, 71
   anatomy of   6
   in anorectal incontinence   41,
      42, 64
   in chronic constipation   43
   in continence   21, 25
   in defaecation   36, 93
   in diabetes   52
   during sleep   20
   electrical stimulation and   160
   exercise training   199
   fibre density   71
   in continence   71, 125
   innervation of   7, 43, 61
   obstetric tears   161
   in pudendal neuropathy   64
   response to rectal distension   72
   in spinal cord lesions   54
   training of   197
   weakness in anorectal
      incontinence   41
Anal sphincter, internal
   anatomy of   6
   in anorectal incontinence   49
   beta-adrenergic relaxation
      of   7
   cause of dysfunction   51
   causes of weakness   72
   childbirth and   44
   in continence   21, 50
   in diabetes   52
   dysfunction in incontinence   50,
      72, 74, 119
   electrical stimulation   89, 160
   in Hirschsprung's disease   106
   loperamide affecting   150
   nerve supply   7
   noradrenaline affecting   51
   parasympathetic nerves   8
   pharmacological abnormalities   51
   pressure   51
   relaxation and sensation   49, 198
   response to distension   35
   resting pressure and   49
   thickness   40
Anal sphincter pressure zone   18
Anal squeeze pressures   6, 21, 64,
      65, 72

after electrical stimulation   160
after postanal repair   162
biofeedback and   158
in continence   46
defaecation and   118
in dementia   118
effect of age on   61
estimation of   131
in faecal impaction   110
in incontinence   46, 71, 72, 112
measurement of   13
mobility and   66
obstetric factors   44, 45
in rectal prolapse   47
in spinal cord lesions   54, 55
Anorectal angle
   age and   67
   in constipation   91
   continence and   22, 111
   in faecal impaction   107, 111
   failure to open   107
   in incontinence   41
   in obstructed defaecation   93
   in perineal descent   46
   restoration of   162
Anorectal function
   age changes in   60–75
   in dementia   117
   faecal impaction and   104
   in faecal incontinence   71–5
   in ulcerative colitis   79
Anorectal incontinence   40–59,
      115, 126
   ageing and   47
   anal reflex in   42
   anal sensation in   47
   anorectal angle in   41
   anorectal sensory loss in   47
   anal sphincter injury causing   40
   biofeedback in   157–8
   cauda equina and   47
   denervation and   41, 42
   EMG studies in   41
   electrical stimulation for   159
   external sphincter in   42, 64
   histological studies   41
   internal sphincter weakness in   49
   latency of anal reflex in   42
   manometry studies   41
   obstetric factors   43
   pelvic floor re-education for   159
   perineal descent in   46
   see also Descending perineal syndrome
   prolapse and   47
   pudendal nerve conduction studies
      in   43
   rectal sensation in   48
   sampling reflex in   48
   single fibre EMG studies   42
   spinal cord disease and   47

surgical treatment 161
treatment of 157–67
Anorectal myomectomy 145
Anorectal pressure 19
Ano-rectal sensation
continence and 22
Anorectal sensory loss 47
Anus
anatomy of 5
lining of 25
motor activity 32
Anxiety reduction 200
Appendicocaecostomy
enema via 164
Aspirin in ulcerative colitis 80
Autonomic degeneration
affecting continence 73
Aversion therapy 183–4
Awareness,
loss of 115

Bacteriuria
incontinence and 125
Behaviour
failure to change 190
Behavioural problems
incontinence and 115, 156
Behavioural therapy 197, 198
failure 188
Bethanecol 8
Bile acids
effect on stools 83, 103
Biofeedback therapy 157–8, 194, 196,
198, 199
assumptions underlying 194
for constipation 158, 197
for irritable bowel syndrome 195
in obstructed defaecation 158
psychological aspects 158
role of 197
Bisacodyl 142
Bladder sensation
constipation and 94
Bladder stimulators 145
Bombesin 8
Bowels
inflammatory disease of 79
Bowel habits
ageing and 60
normal 103
in stroke 121
Bran 140, 141, 187
Bulking agents 140, 187

Campylobacter infection 78
Campylobacter jejuni 79
Cauda equina
anorectal incontinence and 47
internal sphincter and 52
Causes of incontinence 70, 124

Cerebral disease
causing incontinence 114–23,
153–6
Childbirth
pudendal nerve damage from 43
sphincter nerve damage from 43,
44
Children
emotional disturbance in 176
Cholestyramine for diarrhoea 151
Cidapride 143
Cingulate gyrus 3
Clinical assessment 129–32
defaecation history in 129
history taking 129
investigations 131
physical examination 130
Clonidine in diarrhoea 151
Clostridium difficile 78
Codalax 143
Codanthrusate 142
Codeine phosphate for
diarrhoea 149, 150
Cognitive impairment
continence training in 190
incontinence and 192
Colectomy for constipation 144
Colitis
Campylobacter 78
Salmonella 78
ulcerative 79–81
Collection devices 170
Colo-anal anastomosis
effect on recto-anal inhibitory
reflex 35
Colon
anatomy of 3
in defaecation 30
dynamic scintigraphy 30, 31, 88
electrical activity in
constipation 88
faecal loading 88, 154
faecal storage in 32
functional divide 32
irrigation of 137
mass movements in 30
mobility and ageing 61
mobility in constipation 86, 88
muscular activity 4, 61
nerve supply 4
segmented transit studies 87
sympathetic innervation 4
transit through 30
Colonic propulsion 86, 103
Colonometrogram 33
Colorectal cancer 76, 77, 78
Confused patient 180
continence training for 189
Consciousness
impaired 114

Constipation 101–9, 176
  after spinal cord injury 53
  anorectal angle in 91
  as factor in incontinence 178
  biofeedback in treatment 158, 197
  bladder sensation with 94
  causes of 87, 93, 102
  clinical assessment 130
  colonic mobility in 88
  colonic propulsion and 86, 103
  defaecatory difficulty in 91, 104
  definition of 86, 102
  denervation of muscle in 43
  diagnosis of 102
  diet causing 179
  drug-induced 97
  effectiveness of laxatives 143
  electrical activity of colon in 88
  evacuation disturbances 91
  external sphincter in 46
  faecal impaction in 102
  fibre and 139
  gut transit in 86, 103
  gynaecological problems in 95
  haemorrhoids and 96
  hysterectomy as cause 95
  idiopathic *see Idiopathic constipation*
  immobility and 101, 103
  incidence 101
  incontinence secondary to 110–3
  induction of 153
  laxatives as cause 102
  megarectum 94
  in multiple sclerosis 52, 53
  myenteric plexus in 74, 89, 104
  obstructed defaecation in 92, 106
  orocaecal transit times in 90
  pain and 102
  in Parkinson's disease 122
  pathophysiology of 103–7
  psychiatric symptoms 96
  puborectalis muscle in 46
  rectal compliance in 92, 106
  rectal sensation in 93
  role of VIP in 89
  sampling reflex in 92
  small bowel transit in 90
  spinal stimulators for 145
  steroid hormones affecting 96
  stress incontinence with 94
  in stroke patients 121
  substance P in 90
  surgical management 144–5
  urological problems in 94
Continence
  anal cushions in 25
  anal pressure and 22
  anal sensation and 22, 48
  anal sphincter pressure zone
    and 18
  anorectal angle and 22, 111
  external sphincter activity in 21, 25
  flap valve mechanism 22
  internal sphincter in 21, 50
  maintenance of 18–28
  mechanical factors 25
  mucosal component 25
  puborectalis muscle in 22
  rectal pressure and 22, 117
  rectal sensation in 22, 24
  reflex activity and 21
  rectal sensation and 112
  relationship with incontinence 200
  role of sphincters 18, 21, 25, 50, 118
  sampling reflex in 22, 112
  skills involved in 181
  slit-shaped anal canal and 25
  vascular component of 25
Continence training 189
Coprophagia 115
Crohn's disease 82–3

Danthromer 142, 144
Danthron 142
Defaecation 29–39
  act of 36, 114, 117
  ageing and 67
  character of stool and 104
  closing reflex 36
  in constipation 104
  external anal sphincter in 36, 93
  gut transit and 29, 91
  higher control of 3
  history taking 129
  initiation of 29
  intra-abdominal pressure in 36, 106
  intrarectal pressure during 105
  obstructed 92, 106, 145, 158
  patterns of 187
  pelvic floor during 36
  planned 153, 155
  posture of 179
  puborectalis muscle in 93
  quantities of faeces in 37
  rectal activity in 32
  recto-anal inhibitory reflex in 35
  role of colon 30
Dehydration in diarrhoea 149
Dementia 135, 173, 174
  anal resting pressure in 118
  anal squeeze pressures in 118
  anorectal function in 117
  causes of incontinence in 128, 192
  continence training in 189, 191
  faecal incontinence in 128
  faecal loading in 153
  incontinence in 114, 124, 128, 178, 192, 196

pudendal nerve terminal motor
   latency in 119
  rectal contractions in 117
  urinary incontinence 192
Descending perineum syndrome 43,
  46, 49
  examination of 130
  postanal repair and 161
  in rectal intussusception 93
Diabetes mellitus
  anorectal function in 52
  diarrhoea in 73
  incontinence in 52, 72
  pelvic floor neuropathy in 52
Diarrhoea 129
  in AIDS 151
  bile acid 83
  codeine for 149, 150
  collection devices for 170, 171
  in Chrohn's disease 82
  in diabetes 73
  functional 80
  hormone mediated 151
  infective 78
  loperamide for 149
  post vagotomy 150
  spurious 102
  treatment of 149–52
  in ulcerative colitis 79
Diet
  constipation and 179
  effects of 179
  in treatment 187
Dietary fibre
  constipation and 140
  gut transit and 29, 140
Diverticular disease 140, 141
Docusate 142
Dorbanex 143, 144
Duodenum
  Motor activity in 32
Dynamic colonic scintigraphy 30,
  31, 88
Dynamic evacuation
  proctography 93

Electrical stimulation
  in anorectal incontinence 159, 160
Electromyography 15, 41, 42
Emotional experience
  of incontinence 174
Encopresis
  definition 176
  retentive and non-retentive 178
  treatment of 144
Enemas 137
  antegrade 164
  decline in use of 144
  use of 135, 153, 186
Enteric nervous system 8

Enterocolitis 78
Enuresis 178
Ethics of aversion therapy 184
Exercise
  effect on gut transit 30
Exercise programmes in
  treatment 139

Faecal collection devices 170, 171
Faecal impaction
  anal resting pressure in 110
  anorectal angle in 107, 111
  anorectal function and 104
  in constipation 102
  definition 102
  rectal contractions and 105
  rectal sensation in 111
  recto-anal inhibitory reflex in 110
  squeeze pressures in 110
Faecal leakage 111, 126
  containment of 168
Faecal loading 127, 132, 154
  affecting gut transit 90
  characteristics of patients 125
  colonic 88
  constipation and 102
  dietary fibre and 141
  in dementia 153
  Loss of awareness and 115
  in stroke patients 121
  treatment of incontinence
    from 135–48
Faecal smearing 115
Faecal softeners 142
Faeces
  see also Stool
  colonic storage 32
  manual removal of 137
  quantity passed 37
  temperature of 23
Fibre
  effect on gut 29, 140
  effect on stools 103
  incontinence and 154
  in treatment 187
Flap valve theory 22
Flatus
  anal pressure and 23
  distinguished from stool 23
Fluid and electrolyte
  replacement 149
Flutter valve action 25
Food poisoning 78

Gastrocolic reflex 30
  in treatment 187
Golytely 138
Gut brain 5
Gut transit 29, 139
  after treatment 139

age changes   61
assessment of   29
constipation and   103
defaecatory difficulty and   91
dietary fibre and   29
effect of fibre on   140
exercise affecting   30
faecal loading and   90
gynaecological problems and   95
in idiopathic constipation   86
in megarectum   95
nervous control of   89
in Parkinson's disease   90
psychiatric problems and   97
role of activity in   30
role of sigmoid and rectum   104
sex hormones affecting   96
studies of   87

Haemorrhoids and constipation   96
Health problems
   with incontinence   175
Hemiplegia
   rectal contractions in   116
Hirschsprung's disease   35
   see also Megarectum
   caecorectal anastomosis for   145
   constipation in   107
   internal sphincter in   106
   recto-anal inhibitory reflex in   73
   sphincter pressure in   74
   VIP deficiency in   89
Hyperthyroidism
   orocaecal transit time in   91
Hypothalamus
   in control of defaecation   3
Hypothyroidism
   orocaecal transit time in   91
Hysterectomy
   causing constipation   93

Idiopathic constipation   86–100
   colonic abnormalities in   88
   colonic motility in   86
   defaecatory difficulty in   91
   electrical activity of colon in   88
   features of   86
   gynaecological problems in   95
   hysterectomy as cause   95
   megarectum in   94
   myenteric plexus abnormality
      in   89
   obstructed defaecation in   92
   orocaecal transit times in   90
   rectal compliance in   92
   rectal sensation in   93
   small bowel transit time in   90
   stress incontinence and   94
   substance P and VIP in   89, 90
Idiopathic faecal incontinence

   see Anorectal incontinence
Idiopathic intestinal pseudo-
      obstruction   107
Ileo-anal anastomosis   81
Immobility
   constipation and   103
   incontinence and   127
Immunosuppressive drugs
   in Crohn's disease   82
Impaired consciousness
   incontinence during   114
Incidence of incontinence   1
   in residential homes   191
Incontinence
   causes   70, 124
   clinical assessment
      see Clinical assessment
   treatment
      see Treatment
   See also under types
Incontinence laundry service   172
Incontinence pads   168, 169
Infective diarrhoea   78
Inflammatory bowel disease   79
Inflation reflex   21, 72
   absence of   112
Internal sphincterotomy   18
Intestinal mobility   104
   loperamide and   149
Intestinal pseudo-obstruction   107
Intestinal transit
   hormonal effects   96
   in elderly   103
   in idiopathic constipation   90
Intra-abdominal pressure
   in defaecation   36, 106
   effect on anal canal   21
Intractable incontinence
   treatment of   168–72
Investigations   131
Irritable bowel syndrome
   biofeedback therapy   195
Isoprenaline
   effect on sphincter muscle   7

Lactulose   142
Laxatives
   age associated use of   60
   choice of   141
   constipation and   102
   in continence control   155
   effect on stool   102
   effectiveness of   143
   for faecally loaded patient   135
   induced incontinence   112
   osmotic   141
   stimulant   142
   in treatment   186
   use of   141-4
Lazy bowel syndrome   186

Levator ani muscles 6
  in anorectal incontinence 41
  nerve supply 7
Living conditions
  incontinence and 180
Living space
  bowel problems and 180
Loperamide
  effect on anal sphincter 150
  for diarrhoea 149

Manovolumetry 33
Massage in treatment 139, 140
Medication in treatment 185
Megacolon *See* Hirschsprung's *disease*
Megarectum 106
  see also Hirschsprung's disease
  caecorectal anastomosis for 145
  in constipation 94
  definition 94
  sex incidence 95
Melanosis coli
  laxative induced 142
Meningocele 8
Menopause
  anal squeeze pressures and 65
Mental health
  incontinence and 175
Mental well-being
  effect of incontinence on 174,
    175, 176
Methylcellulose
  effects of 140
Micro-enema 135
  for faecal loading 154
Micturition
  anal canal pressure during 20
Migrating motor complexes 19
Mini Mental Status Exam 192
Mobility 130
  defaecation and 180
  incontinence and 125
Motility
  in Parkinson's disease 122
  squeeze pressure and 66
Multifactorial causes of
    incontinence 134
Multi-infarct disease 114
Multiple sclerosis 52, 195, 197
Multivariate analysis
  of incontinent patients 125–6
Muscle
  age affecting 62
Muscle sling 6
Myelomeningocele 198
Myenteric degeneration
  senna and 142
Myenteric plexus
  abnormality of 89, 104, 106
  in constipation 74, 104

integrity of 73

Nerve conduction velocity
  age changes 64
Neurogenic faecal incontinence 40,
    115
Neuropeptides
  regulatory 5, 8
  see also specific substances
Neuropeptide Y 5, 8
Nocturnal enuresis 178
Noradrenaline
  effect on sphincter muscle 7
  sphincter sensitivity to 51

Obstetrics
  anorectal incontinence and 43
  sphincter damage and 43, 44, 45
Occult blood tests 77
Ondansetron 151
Orocaecal transit 90
  loperamide affecting 150

Pain
  constipation and 102
Paraplegia
  constipation in 143
  continence in 48
  incontinence in 197
  rectal contractions in 116
  recto-anal reflex in 65
Parkinson's disease 90, 122
Pelvic floor
  abnormal descent of 46, 51
  anatomy of 6
  denervation 43
  in diabetes 52
  during defaecation 36
  hormonal changes and 65
  nerve supply 6
  physiotherapy for 159
  re-education of 159
  surgery for constipation 145
  weakness in incontinence 41
Perianal sutures 164
Perineal descent 43, 44, 46, 49
  examination of 130
  in rectal intussusception 93
  postanal repair and 163
Perineal nerves
  injury to 43
Peristalsis
  substance P and 5
Personal experience of
  incontinence 174
Personality
  disturbances 176
  incontinence and 175
Phosphate enemas 135
Physical abuse

resulting from incontinence   176
Physical examination of patient   130
Physiotherapy
    for pelvic floor muscles   159
Phytobezoars   187
Picolax   137, 139, 155
Polyuria
    nocturnal   169
Postanal repair   41, 50, 161
    aims of   162
    results of   162
Post defaecation reflex   36
Posture for defaecation   179
Predefaecation urge   186
Proctectomy
    effect on recto-anal inhibitory
        reflex   35
Prostitis   79
Proctocolectomy   81
Proctometrogram   33
Prompted voiding and drinking
    procedure   189
Propranolol   7
Pseudomembraneous colitis   78
Psychiatric symptoms
    in constipation   96
Psycho-analytic approach to
    treatment   182
Psychological approach to
    treatment   177
Psychological aspects of
    biofeedback   158
    incontinence   173–207
Psychological assessment of
    patient   178
Puborectalis muscle   6
    activity   18
    in anorectal incontinence   41
    in continence   22
    in defaecation   93
    nerve supply   7
Pudendal nerve   6
    in anorectal incontinence   43
    damage from straining   46
    entrapment   43
    injury to 44, 161
    obstetric damage to   43
Pudendal nerve terminal motor
    latency   43, 64
    age changes   64
    in constipation   46
    in dementia   119
    in incontinence   72
    obstetric factors   43
    in prolapse   47
    in straining   46
Pudendal neuropathy   46, 64, 127
    in dementia   119
    detection   64
    in incontinence   71, 72

Pudendal sensory responses   120
Purgation   61

Rectal activity
    in defaecation   32
    measurement   92
Rectal anterial wall
    prolapse of   93
Rectal balloon distension
    in biofeedback   158
Rectal bleeding   76, 130
Rectal carcinoma   79, 170
Rectal compliance   92
    after hysterectomy   96
    in constipation   106
    in spinal cord injury   54
Rectal contractions
    in continence and
        incontinence   118
    following distension   33, 105, 117
    impaction and   105
    normal   116
    uninhibited   116, 127
Rectal distension
    contraction following   33, 105, 117
    effect on anal sphincters   21, 35, 72
    loss of awareness of   115
    response to   32, 50
    sensory and reflex responses   34
    sphincter response to   112
    in spinal cord injury   54
Rectal examination   132
Rectal function
    assessment   33
    See also Anorectal function
Rectal motility
    cerebral control of   116
    in cerebral disease   116
    hypertonic   106
Rectal motor complexes   32, 92
Rectal pressure   117
    in continence and
        incontinence   22, 117
Rectal prolapse   47, 49, 163
Rectal response
    phases of   33
Rectal sensation   8, 198
    in anorectal incontinence   48
    after hysterectomy   96
    age affecting   65
    assessment of   92, 93
    in constipation   93
    in continence   24, 112
    in diabetes   52
    in faecal impaction   111
    in incontinence   74
    sacral cord and 94
Rectal sensory neuropathy   94
Recto-anal inhibitory reflex   14, 73
    ageing and   65

in defaecation   35
in faecal impaction   106, 110
in Hirschsprung's disease   73
in megarectum   95
myenteric plexus and   35
Rectocele   93
Rectopexy   163
Rectosigmoid motility   30
Rectum
  anatomy of   5
  contractile activity   32
  delayed filling   92
  in delayed gut transit   104
  manovolumetry   33
  motility studies   32, 105
  motor activity   32
  mucosal electro-sensitivity   94
  nerve supply   4
  response to distension   32
  smooth muscle of   6
  unstable   116
Recurrence of incontinence   139
Residential care institutions   178
  incidence of incontinence in   155,
    191
  staff training in   193
Retentive and non-retentive
  encopresis   178
Reward and punishment techniques
  of treatment   183–5

Sacral cord dysfunction   94
Salazopyrine   82
Salicylate in ulcerative colitis   80
Salmonella infection   78
Salmonella enteritidis   78
Salmonella typhimurium   78
Sampling reflex
  in constipation   92
  continence and   22, 112
  in incontinence   48
  temperature and   23
Scybala   102
Senna   142
Sex hormones
  effect on bowel function   96
Sham sensory retraining   199
Sigmoid colon
  in delayed gut transit   104
  motility   87
Sigmoid volvulus   187
Sleep
  sphincter activity in   20
Social aspects of incontinence   174
Sodium picosulphate 139, 142, 155
  see also Picolax
Somatostatin   8, 151
Spina bifida   195
Spinal stimulators for
    constipation   145

Sphincterotomy   18
Spinal cord disease
  anorectal incontinence in   47
  incontinence in   53–5
Spinal cord injury
  constipation following   53
  incontinence in   53–5
  urinary incontinence following   53
Steroids
  in ulcerative colitis   80
Stimulus control in treatment   187
Stool
  see also Faeces
  bile acids affecting   103
  character of   104
  consistency of   111, 154, 157
  distinguished from flatus   23
  effect of laxatives on   102
  fibre intake affecting   103
Straining at stool
  constipation and   101
  diet and   179
  pudendal nerve damage from   46
Stress incontinence   94, 159, 198
Strokes
  constipation in   121
  incontinence and   114, 121–2
Substance P   5, 8
  in chronic constipation   90
  in ulcerative colitis   79
  peristalsis and   5
Substance PYY   8
Sulphasalazine   80
Suppositories   135, 186
  shape and insertion   137, 138
Symptomatic incontinence
    76–85

Tabes dorsalis   18
Temperature
  ano-rectal sensation and   22
Terminal reservoir syndrome   104
Terminology of incontinence   175
Toilets
  access to   180, 181
  design of   179
Toilet sitting
  prompted   187
Treatment of incontinence 133–4,
    135–48
  anal sphincter training   197
  anorectal incontinence   157–67
  anxiety reduction   200
  aversive consequences   183–4
  behavioural approach to   182
  behavioural therapy   197, 198
  biofeedback in   194, 196, 197,
    198, 199
  continence training   189
  electrical astimulation in   159

enemas and suppositories in   186
incontinence secondary to cerebral
    disease   153–6
initial failure   137
inpatient or outpatient   185
intractable incontinence   168–72
laxatives in   186
medication in   185
planned defaecation   153, 155
prompted voiding and drinking
    procedure   189
psycho-analytical approach   182
psychological approach   177
recurrence after   139
results   160, 196
reward and punishment
    techniques   183–5
secondary to faecal loading   135–48
sham sensory retraining   199
simple measures   133
stimulus control in   187
stress incontinence   198
use of diet   187
use of gastrocolic reflex   187

use of massage   139, 140
Ulcerative colitis   79–81
Uninhibited neurogenic bladder   117
Urinary drainage system   170
Urinary incontinence
    after spinal injury   53
    behavioural approach to   182
    in dementia   192
    electrical stimulation for   159
    management of   169–70
    personal experience of   174
    psychological aspects   173
    treatment   190

Vagus nerve   4
Vasoactive intestinal peptide   5, 8
    in colonic nerve fibres   89
    in constipation   89
    in Hirschsprung's disease   89
VIPomas   151

Wheat bran   140
Wheelchairs and toilets   180